WELLNESS COUNCIL OF A

Walking4 WELLNESS

FOUR SIMPLE STEPS TO ACHIEVE YOUR BEST BODY AND LIFE

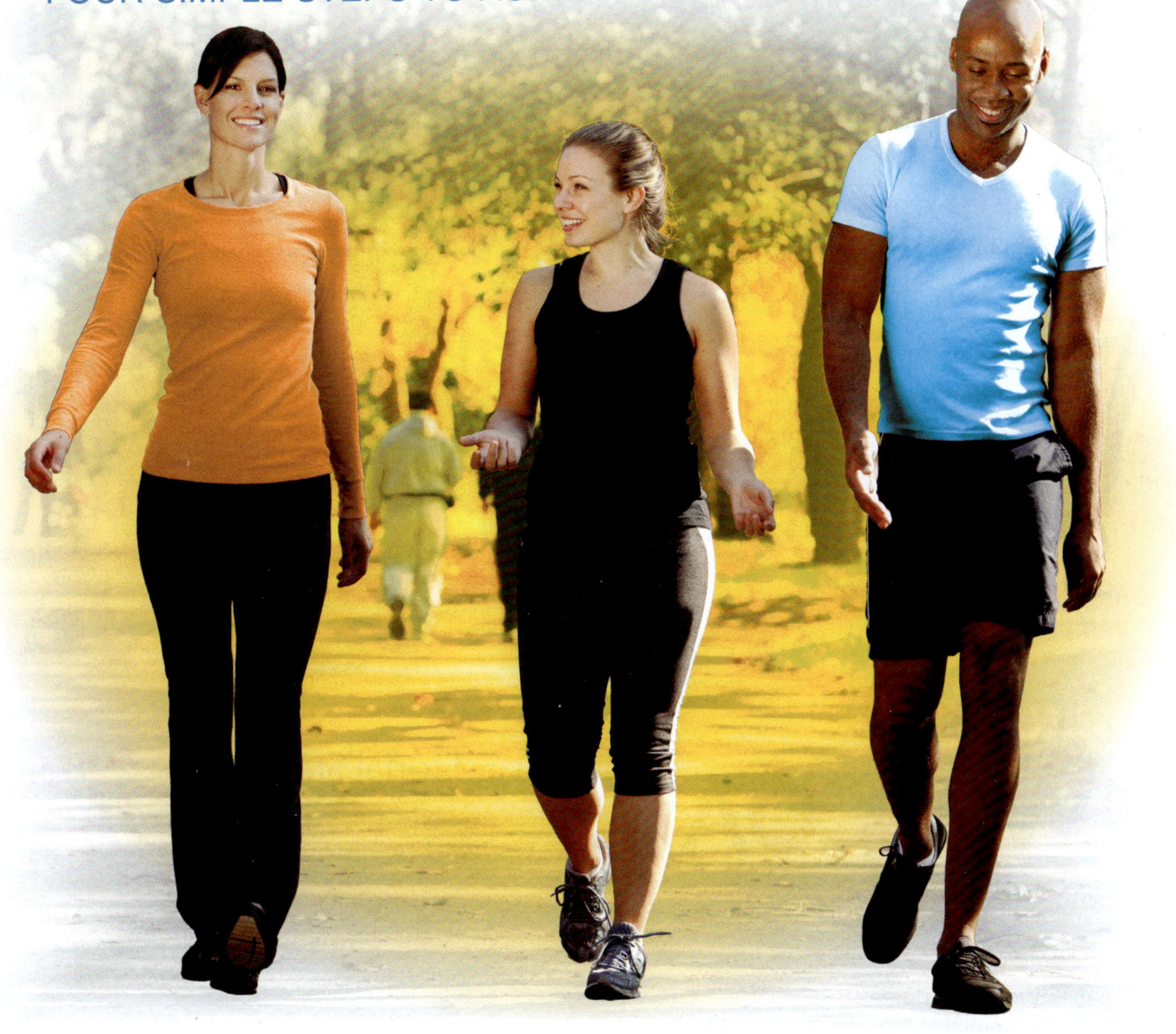

About WELCOA

The Wellness Council of America (WELCOA) was established as a national not-for-profit organization in the mid 1980s through the efforts of a number of forward-thinking business and health leaders. Drawing on the vision originally set forth by William Kizer, Sr., Chairman Emeritus of Central States Indemnity, and WELCOA founding Directors that included Dr. Louis Sullivan, former Secretary of Health and Human Services, and Warren Buffett, Chairman of Berkshire Hathaway, WELCOA has helped influence the face of workplace wellness in the U.S.

Today, WELCOA has become one of the most respected resources for workplace wellness in America. With a membership in excess of 5,000 organizations, WELCOA is dedicated to improving the health and well-being of all working Americans. Located in America's heartland, WELCOA makes its national headquarters in one of America's healthiest business communities—Omaha, Nebraska.

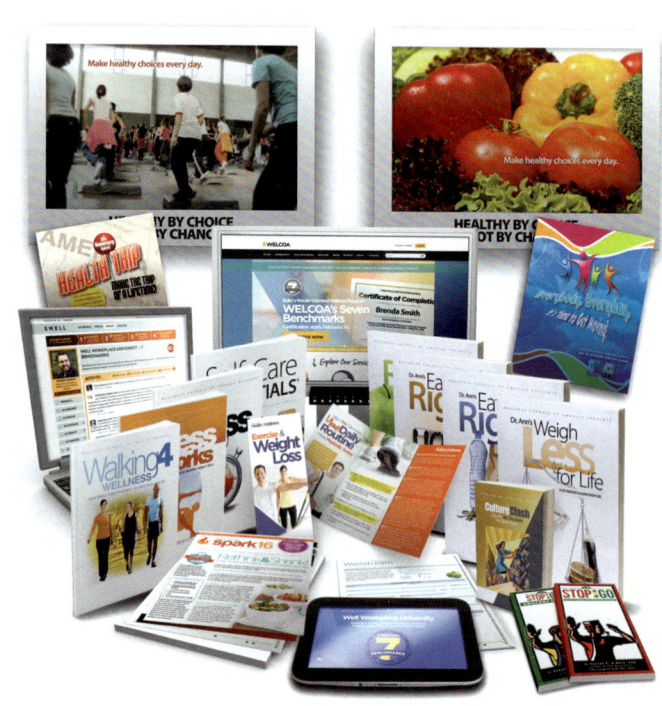

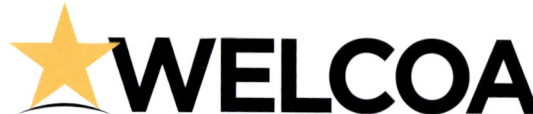

17002 Marcy Street, Suite 140 | Omaha, NE 68118
PH: 402-827-3590 | FX: 402-827-3594 | welcoa.org

Editorial Staff

Author:	Sean Foy, MA
Executive Editor:	David Hunnicutt, PhD
Managing Editor:	Brittanie Leffelman, MS
Contributing Editors:	Carie Maguire
Multimedia Designer:	Adam Paige

Table Of
Contents

About Sean Foy 4

Foreword by Dr. David Hunnicutt 5

Our Walking 4 Wellness Dream 6

Introduction: Mirror, Mirror On The Wall 8

Chapter 1: Four Simples Steps To Walk This Way 12

Chapter 2: Walking 4 Your Body 30

Chapter 3: Walking 4 Your Mind 50

Chapter 4: Walking 4 Your Career & Finances 66

Chapter 5: Walking 4 Your Heart & Spirit 80

Chapter 6: Walking 4 Living Well 96

Chapter 7: Win 4 Today—Putting It All Together 104

In Summary: Walking 4 Wellness 110

About
Sean Foy ma

Sean Foy, MA, is an internationally renowned authority on fitness, weight management and healthy living. As an author, exercise physiologist, behavioral coach and speaker, Sean has earned the reputation as "America's Fast Fitness Expert." With an upbeat, positive and sensible approach to making fitness happen, even with the busiest of schedules, he has taken his message of "simple moves" fitness all over the world.

Sean is the author of the Wellness Council of America flag ship physical activity book, *Fitness That Works: Simple Moves To Make Exercise Happen Between 9-5*, as well as *The 10 Minute Total Body Breakthrough* and the co-creator of an award winning children's health and fitness program, *LEAN KIDS*. Foy is the author and developer of the signature fitness program for The Biggest Loser® Pro Training program. He has also partnered with New York Times best selling authors, Rick Warren, Dr. Mark Hyman and Dr. Daniel Amen in the authoring, development and creation of a faith-based global wellness initiative called, "The Daniel Plan." Among numerous other awards, he received the "Nike Go" Top National Health Education Program Award and the California Governor Health Educator of the Year Award.

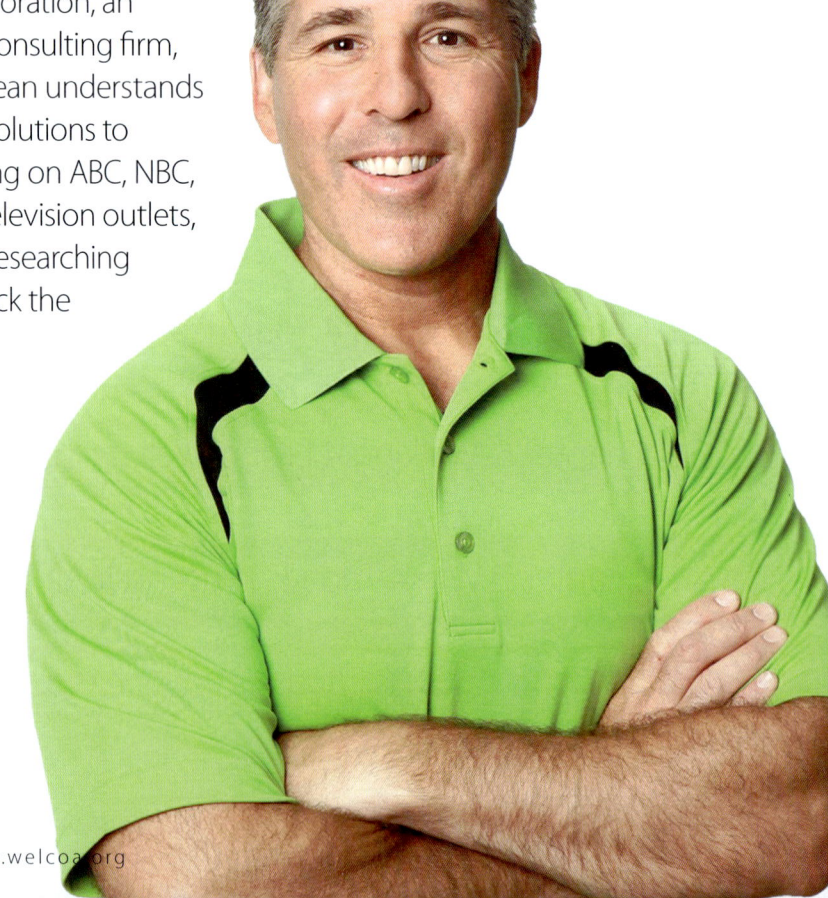

As a husband and father of two, as well as President and founder of Personal Wellness Corporation, an international wellness education and consulting firm, and **www.wintodaywellness.com**, Sean understands "busy" and brings his real life exercise solutions to audiences wherever he goes. Appearing on ABC, NBC, FOX, CBS and other popular national television outlets, he has spent the last 20 years testing, researching and sharing his findings on how to crack the code to make fitness work.

Sean has helped thousands of individuals all over the world with their wellness needs as an author, personal trainer, counselor, presenter and business owner and is committed to encouraging everyone to attain optimal well-being for body, mind and spirit!

Foreword
David Hunnicutt phd

There's magic in this book.

In fact, it's magic of the most powerful kind. It's the kind of magic that has the power to change your life for the better. It's the kind of magic that will put years in your life and life in your years.

And it's not a pipe dream.

If you heed the advice presented in this book, your life will change—and it will change for the better. And there's a mountain of research to back it up.

Indeed, if there's anything that we know about improving health, it's this: one of the greatest predictors of sickness and death is a low fitness level. By following the simple recommendations put forth in this book, you will not only improve your health status but you will improve the overall quality of your life as well.

Indeed, if you want to get the most juice for the squeeze from your life, then walking has to be a part of it.

To lead the journey, I've called on my great friend and colleague— Sean Foy—to help you take your health to the next level. In fact, Sean Foy is one of the nation's leading experts on the power of physical activity. In this book, Sean will help you to harness the power of walking—and he'll do it in a way that's safe, productive and FUN.

It's been said that every great journey begins with the first step. In this case, it's literally true. And by taking that first step, you are beginning a journey that will result in profound changes—changes that will allow you to take advantage of all the opportunities that are ahead of you.

Congratulations on stepping it up, you are in for the trip of a lifetime—and Sean Foy is the perfect person to lead your journey.

Warmest Regards,

David Hunnicutt, PhD
CEO
Wellness Council of America

About **Dr. Hunnicutt**

Since his arrival at WELCOA in 1995, David Hunnicutt, PhD has developed countless publications that have been widely adopted in businesses and organizations throughout North America. Known for his ability to make complex issues easier to understand, David has a proven track-record of publishing health and wellness material that helps employees lead healthier lifestyles. David travels extensively advocating better health practices and radically different thinking in organizations of all kinds.

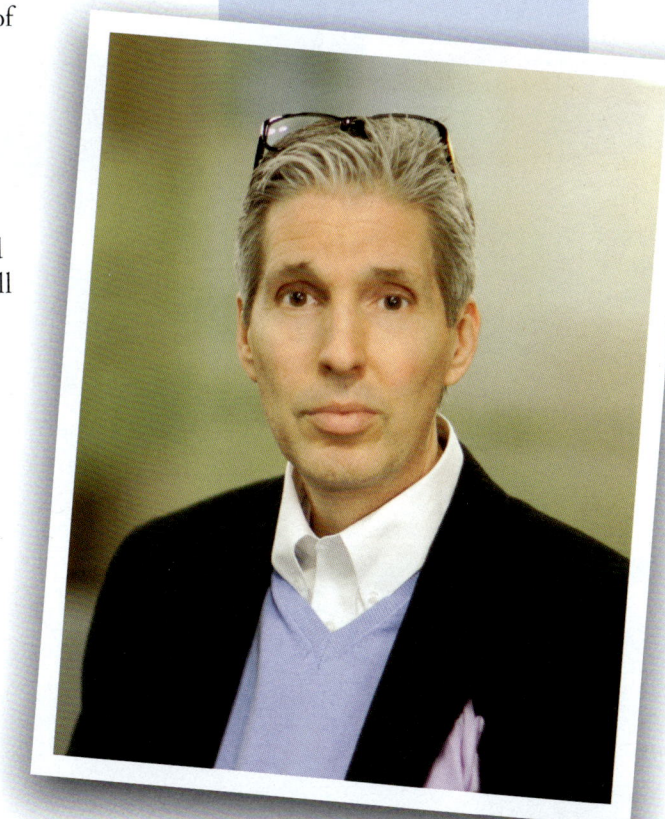

Our Walking4Wellness Dream

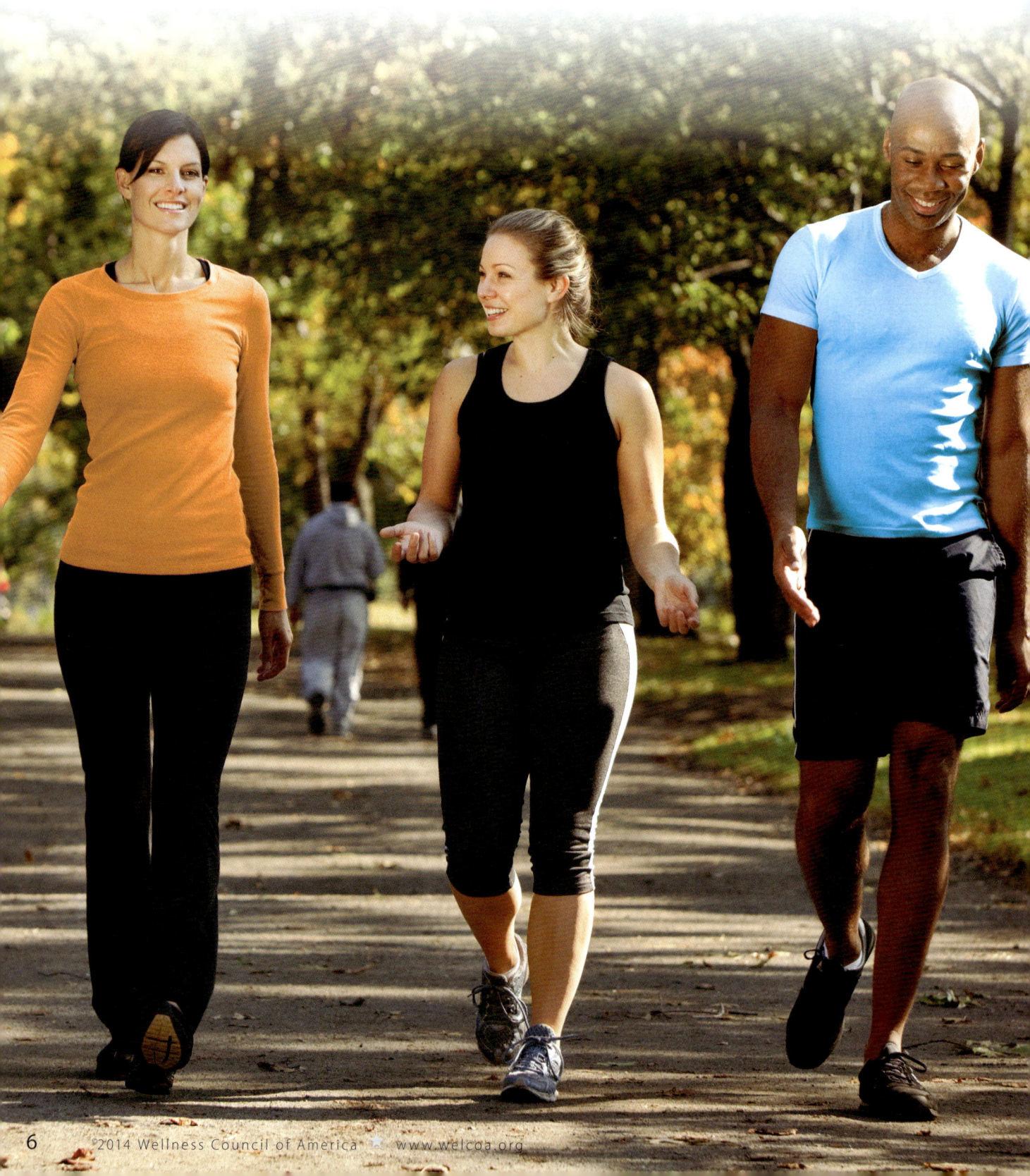

From the Tread of Sean Foy...

WELCOA and I had a dream when writing this book.

We dreamt of you, your family, your company and your community realizing optimal health and wellness for body, heart, mind and spirit.

We saw a clear vision of hundreds of thousands of people, like you, all across the country walking with energy, strength, happiness, health, passion, purpose and experiencing the joy and health of moving.

We strongly believe, by putting into action the steps found in this book, you will discover a proven path to realize your personal health and wellness dreams for your very best life.

We want you to know we will be with you every step of the way, encouraging, instructing, challenging and dreaming right along with you.

So let's get to it...Here's to your dreams!

Sean

Introduction

Mirror Mirror
ON THE WALL…

The only real conflict you will ever have in your life won't be with others but with yourself.

SHANNON L. ALDER

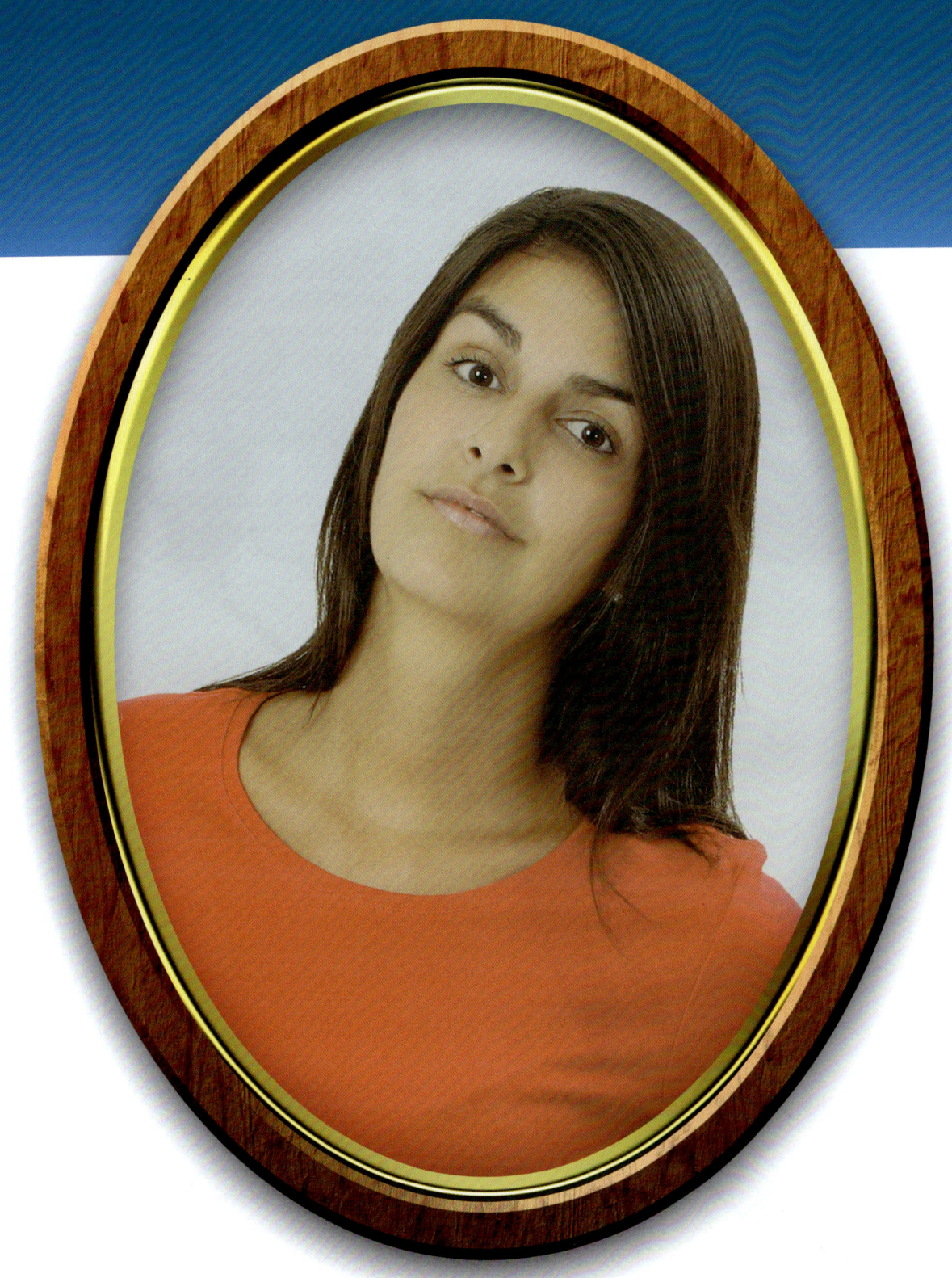

Mirror Mirror
ON THE WALL…

Do you remember the famous fairy tale, Snow White? Do you also remember the popular scene when Snow White's nemesis, the wicked, but beautiful queen stood before her reflection, melodiously inquiring, "Mirror, mirror on the wall…who's the fairest of them all?" And without fail and on queue, the magical mirror responded: "You my Queen are the fairest of all." The Queen was always pleased with the Magic Mirror's response…until the day Snow White arrived on the scene. Talk about "a game changer!"

What about you? Imagine you were to stand in front of a magical mirror. Only this one is a "Wellness Mirror" designed to help you see the truth about your current and future health, fitness, finances, relationships, career and life. Go ahead, take a peek…

✓ What do you see?

✓ How do you feel?

✓ What are your thoughts?

Whatever images may appear for you with this quick glimpse, you'll be excited to know this book, *Walking 4 Wellness*, will help you transform the way you look and feel with four simple steps you can take today to achieve your very best body and life!

Peak Wellness

Unlike other fitness or wellness books, *Walking 4 Wellness* takes the most popular form of exercise in the world, walking, and shows you step by step how to make daily positive strides to reach your summit of optimal health, wellness and ultimately how to realize the life you've always desired.

All of us dream about a life filled with vibrant physical health, meaningful work, close relationships, financial security and a sense of meaning and purpose—but rarely attain it. According to global research, only 7% of us are actually thriving in each of these areas, obtaining what I like to call "Peak Wellness." Can you relate? Do you feel the same way? Maybe you've lost 15 pounds and gained

20 back. Or maybe you've been trying to get out of debt for some time now, but something always seems to get in the way. If you frequently feel like you've been taking two steps forward but then three steps back, you are not alone and I've got good news. With this trusted guide, you'll discover a four-step walking and wellness plan used by countless others who have successfully reached their peak and want to show you how you can do it too!

Are you interested in losing weight or reducing stress or increasing your energy level? In the following chapters you'll discover tried and true "walking paths" with detailed "markers" placed by successful travelers before you, designed to help you reach your personal goals and wellness peak.

Right from the beginning of this book, you will have the opportunity to determine and select your personal "path" with your Walking 4 Wellness assessment. This tool will allow you to identify wellness priorities for your body, mind, career, relationships and spirit.

You will discover the best walking plans to:

✓ Melt off body fat, lose weight and keep it off

✓ Rev up your energy

✓ Break through stress

✓ Boost your mood

✓ Improve your creativity

✓ Increase your earning potential

✓ Enhance your love life

✓ Tone and tighten your entire body

Whether you choose to select one or all of the Walking 4 Wellness paths, you'll be provided with a customized and flexible 4, 8, 12 or 16-week walking program designed to help you reach your personal wellness goals. Regardless of your starting point, by the end of your program you'll be prepared to celebrate your successes by completing a 5K, 10K or ½ marathon challenge, if you'd like.

Whatever your goal may be—whether it's weight loss, stress management or completing a 5K or ½ marathon event, you'll see how walking can dramatically impact not only your physical fitness and health, but also everything else in your life, like your:

✓ Relationships

✓ Work

✓ Aging

✓ Memory

✓ Happiness

✓ Productivity

✓ Finances

✓ Faith

✓ Passion

✓ Purpose

…and so much more.

With this trusted guide, you'll discover a four-step walking and wellness plan used by countless others who have successfully reached their peak and want to show you how you can do it too!

With each chapter, you'll uncover proven tips, techniques and strategies you can use today—right now—to help you reach your peak and maximize your desired results.

I'll also be sharing proven resources that will aid you in your journey which you can incorporate into your walking program and daily life.

Lastly, you'll be motivated and guided by four simple steps throughout this book and introduced to individuals who are using them to successfully Walk 4 Wellness and you'll quickly see how you can do it too!

I promise you, by following *Walking 4 Wellness* and the simple steps found in this book, you'll be able to look in the mirror, smile and be very happy about the way you look and feel! Are you ready?

Walk this way…

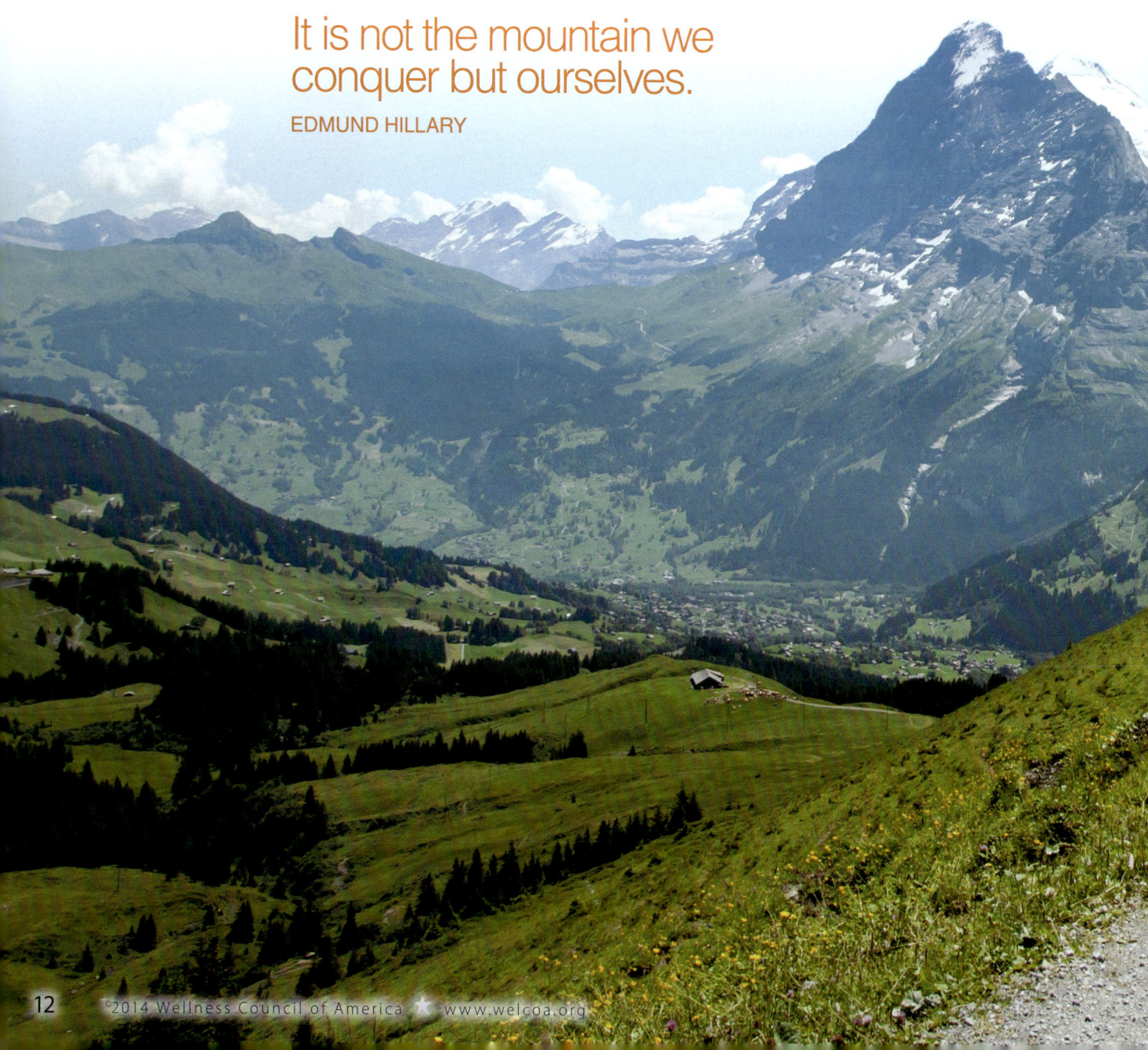

Chapter 1

Four Simple Steps To
Walk This Way

It is not the mountain we conquer but ourselves.

EDMUND HILLARY

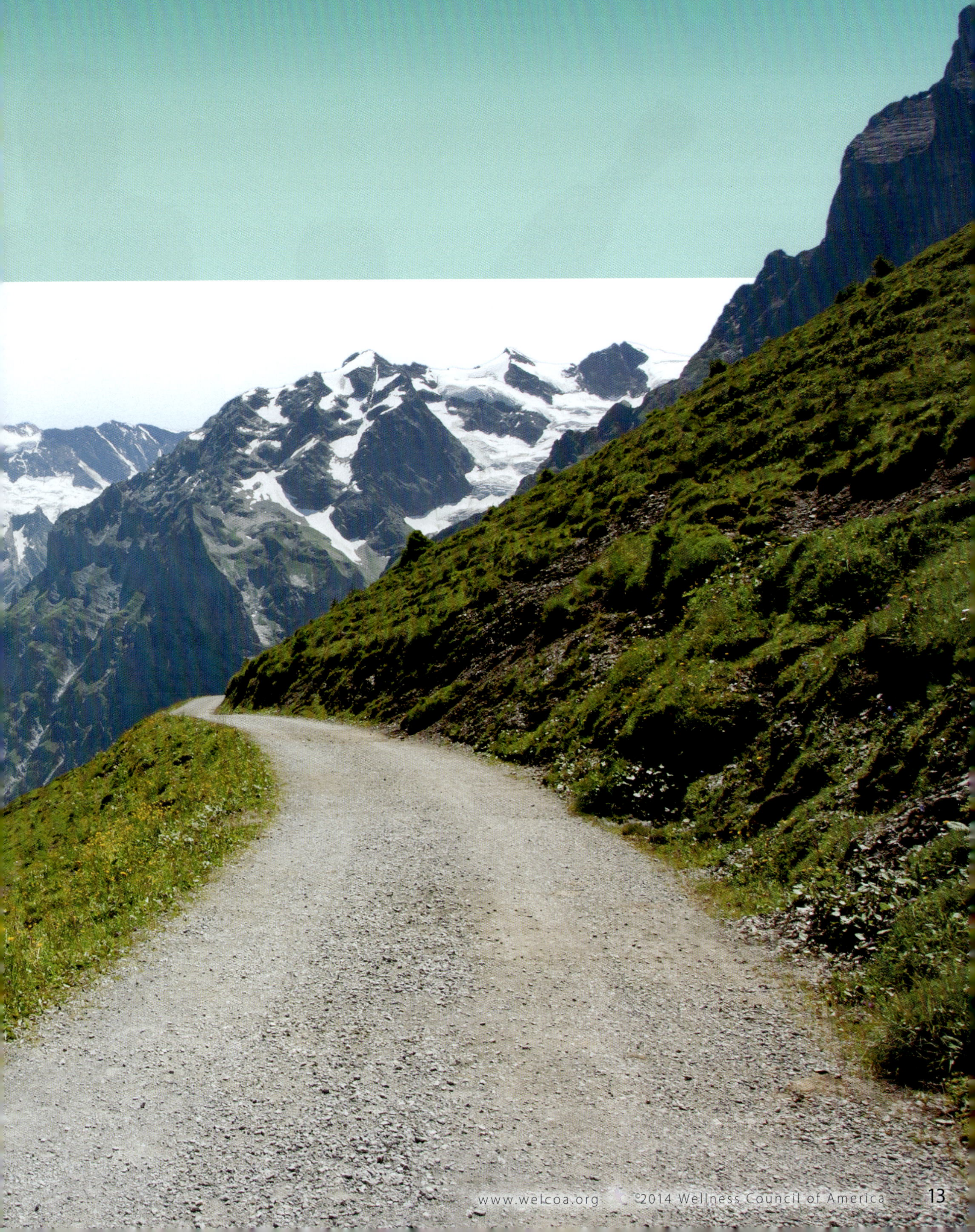

Four Simple Steps To
Walk This Way

Meet You At The Top!

Who would have thought it possible? Yuichiro Muira, now into his seventies, dreamt of one day reaching the summit of Mount Everest. Gone were the days of his youth when he was a healthy and fit alpine skier and daredevil. Since his retirement, Muira had endured two heart surgeries, had become out of shape and overweight leaving many, including some of his closest family members to think he was crazy. Determined to recapture the joy of his youth and his dream, Muira set out walking every day in the city streets of Tokyo. Gaining confidence and strength, he used a pack fastened to his back, replacing the weight he was losing with added weights. He then added ankle weights to his walks and progressed to hiking and climbing local hills and then smaller mountains. Now with a newfound fitness, strength, endurance, passion and purpose, Yuichiro Muira successfully reached his ultimate dream of becoming the oldest person, at the age of 80, to scale to the summit of Mount Everest! He has been quoted as saying, "It is important to have a dream no matter how old you are." The great news is Muira has a lot to look forward to as well—you see—his father skied down the face of the Alps at the young age of 99!

How about you? What are your dreams? What or where is your peak? What are your goals? You may think yourself too old, too out of shape, too busy, too lazy, too whatever, I am here to tell you it is never too late! I am excited to share with you in this chapter, and throughout this book four simple and proven steps Yuichiro Muira and countless others have successfully mastered to help them Walk 4 Wellness and reach their peak.

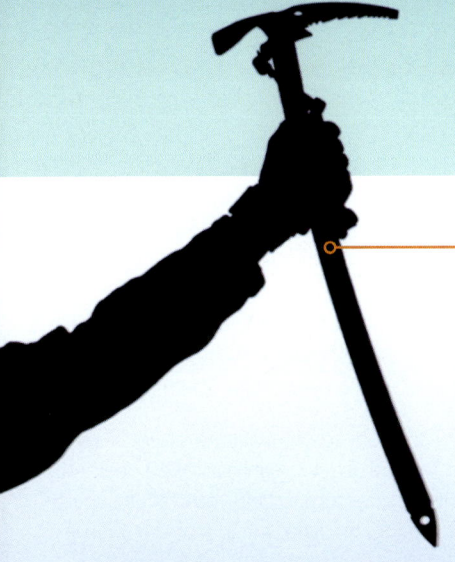

You may think yourself too old, too out of shape, too busy, too lazy, too whatever, I am here to tell you it is never too late!

We will explore:

✓ Walking 4 Wellness: An Overview Of Steps 1-4

✓ Step 1—Think Well: Ask The Right Questions

   a. Your Walking 4 Wellness Assessment

   b. Your top Priorities

✓ Step 2—Plan Well: Casting Your Vision

   a. Determining Your Destination

   b. Setting Your Goals

   c. Selecting Your Path

You Can Do This!

That day, Doreen's life would never be the same. She came into the health club I was working in at the time and shared with me, "Sean, I've got to make a change!" Doreen, a single middle-aged mother of two boys had spent her life pouring her love and devotion into her boys while managing a home as well as working full time as a hair stylist and thought it was about time she took some much needed time and attention for herself. "Sean, I've gained 30 pounds over the last 20 years, my blood pressure is sky high and my cholesterol is over the top. My doctor is bugging me all the time to start exercising. I know it's time for me to make some changes—I just don't know where to begin." I smiled and told Doreen, "Today, you are taking your first step to your new fit and healthy future." We talked for a while about her dreams, goals and plans and then walked over to the treadmill area and I showed her how to safely start, stop and increase the speed and elevation of the machine. I could see she was a little hesitant and timid at first. But, after a couple of minutes of light walking I could see her confidence increasing. A British citizen, still with a strong British accent, Doreen, looked down at her feet and up at me with a glimmer of hope in her eyes and a smile on her face and said, "This is lovely. I can do this!" Indeed she can! Doreen has been faithfully walking and working out over the last 30 years since that visit. How do I know? Doreen is my mother! She is now in her mid 80's and is more fit today than she was when she was in her 40's! I am proud to say, Doreen (my mom), is an amazing example of how powerful Walking 4 Wellness can be. In the words of my mother, "This is lovely— You can do this too!" Join my mom and countless others who have taken that first step and are Walking 4 Wellness, not looking back and are reaping the benefits of a healthy, fit and happy life.

Now It's Time To Learn How To Use This Book With An Overview Of The 4 Steps

Four Simple Steps To Walk This Way

Walking 4 Wellness: An Overview Of Steps 1–4

Throughout this book you'll be introduced to four steps—steps my mother used to walk towards her best life and Yuichiro used to scale Mount Everest at 80 years old. These steps will become trusted markers along your journey to help you reach your destination. I encourage you to take a moment to review the four steps below.

1 **Think Well: Ask The Right Questions.** In this chapter and throughout this book you'll be introduced to crucial and essential questions others who have successfully reached their wellness peak have asked and answered. First you'll get a chance to take a peek into your wellness by completing your Walking 4 Wellness assessment that will provide you with a list of questions to help you identify where your current wellness for your body, mind, career/finances, relationships and spirit journey is beginning. You'll be able to score your results as well as reassess your progress.

2 **Plan Well: Casting Your Vision—Determining Your Destination.** We will show you how to improve your Walking 4 Wellness scores by "Vision Casting" and turning your dreams into action. In this step we will show you how to set specific and concrete goals to put you on your path.

3 **Walk Well: Proven Paths To Get You Where You Want To Be.** We will unfold for you detailed walking plans others have successfully used to help you significantly improve your designated area of interest for:

✓ Walking 4 Your Body
✓ Walking 4 Your Mind
✓ Walking 4 Your Career & Finances
✓ Walking 4 Your Heart & Spirit

4 **Live Well: Tips, Resources And Strategies To Keep You Moving.** We will provide you with tips, resources and suggestions to help you stay on top and keep on moving! Finally, we will help you design your Walking 4 Wellness plan. You will be able to create a 4, 8, 12 or 16 week walking plan focusing on your wellness needs by putting all of the four steps together into your own personal plan of action.

1 Think Well: Ask The Right Questions

Imagine you are standing in front of your "Wellness Mirror" again and now you are going to take a closer look at where you are today. In a moment I'll be asking you a number of questions to help you take an honest look at your body, mind, career and finances, and heart and spirit. The goal of Walking 4 Wellness is to help you thrive in each of the four areas. To assist you in your journey, we will take our first step by taking a closer look "in the mirror" at your current wellness status. But before you do, I'd like you to promise me you'll do two things as you answer each question:

1. **Don't beat yourself up.** Asking questions about your health and wellness can feel a little overwhelming. As you are completing your assessment remember to be kind to yourself. Yes, be honest, as it is important to understand where you currently are before you can establish where you want to be, but be sure to do it constructively and kindly.

2. **Remember to smile.** To help you accomplish Step #1 and ease any potential discomfort, I frequently encourage my clients to smile as they complete their assessment. I know it may seem silly, but it helps remind us to give ourselves a break. Regardless, remember to give yourself plenty of grace and try not to be critical, be honest, but don't be harsh with yourself.

Take a moment to look closely in the "mirror" by completing the following Walking 4 Wellness assessment on the next page. Please circle the response most appropriate for you next to each question. At the end of each section, total your scores.

Walking 4 Wellness Assessment

BODY	Rarely	Sometimes	Frequently	Always
1 I am physically active, exercising on a regular basis to improve my health, strength, endurance and flexibility.	1	2	3	4
2 I consider my physical fitness to be good to excellent.	1	2	3	4
3 I maintain a healthy and desirable weight.	1	2	3	4
4 I feel good about my appearance and the condition of my body.	1	2	3	4
5 I choose healthy, nutritious foods restoring my body and health.	1	2	3	4
6 I sleep seven to eight hours each night.	1	2	3	4
7 I have an abundance of energy throughout the day.	1	2	3	4
8 My body is free from pain.	1	2	3	4
9 My body is free from disease.	1	2	3	4
10 I have annual medical and dental checkups.	1	2	3	4
Add up your scores in each column:				
Add up all columns for your total score for BODY:				

MIND	Rarely	Sometimes	Frequently	Always
1 I manage my stress well by choosing positive outlets such as relaxation through exercise, hobbies, time with others, etc.	1	2	3	4
2 I can recognize and express my emotions and needs well.	1	2	3	4
3 I speak positively to myself.	1	2	3	4
4 I set realistic goals and expectations of myself.	1	2	3	4
5 I feel I am responsible and have considerable control over my life.	1	2	3	4
6 I learn or do something interesting every day.	1	2	3	4
7 I find ways to enjoy today—rarely worrying about tomorrow.	1	2	3	4
8 I find happiness and joy in living.	1	2	3	4
9 When I am angry or upset I share my feelings in constructive ways with others.	1	2	3	4
10 In general, I feel happy and satisfied with my life.	1	2	3	4
Add up your scores in each column:				
Add up all columns for your total score for MIND:				

CAREER & FINANCES	Rarely	Sometimes	Frequently	Always
1 I am happy and fulfilled in my present job or career.	1	2	3	4
2 I find what I do in my work is challenging and rewarding.	1	2	3	4
3 I am presently using my skills and talents in a productive and meaningful way with my work.	1	2	3	4
4 I am regularly proactive, challenging myself to learn something new to advance my career opportunities.	1	2	3	4
5 I am hopeful and excited about my future career opportunities.	1	2	3	4
6 I am satisfied with my present standard of living.	1	2	3	4
7 I am confident I have enough money to do what I want to do in life.	1	2	3	4
8 I have the knowledge and skills I need to manage my money well and meet my present financial obligations.	1	2	3	4
9 I follow a financial budget.	1	2	3	4
10 I am hopeful about my financial future.	1	2	3	4
Add up your scores in each column:				
Add up all columns for your total score for CAREER & FINANCES:				

HEART & SPIRIT	Rarely	Sometimes	Frequently	Always
1 I have close and fulfilling relationships in my life.	1	2	3	4
2 I resolve conflict with others in a productive way.	1	2	3	4
3 I have someone in my life I can talk to about my private life.	1	2	3	4
4 I consider the feelings of others and choose my relationships based on mutual kindness and respect.	1	2	3	4
5 I forgive others when wronged and do not hold resentment or bitterness towards others.	1	2	3	4
6 I have a meaningful spiritual or religious practice in my life.	1	2	3	4
7 I believe my life has an important purpose and/or meaning.	1	2	3	4
8 I am satisfied with my spiritual life.	1	2	3	4
9 I engage in acts of caring, good will and charity towards others.	1	2	3	4
10 I look for ways to help others in need.	1	2	3	4
Add up your scores in each column:				
Add up all columns for your total score for HEART & SPIRIT:				

Four Simple Steps To Walk This Way

Walking 4 Wellness Priorities

SCORES AT A GLANCE

Congratulations! Now that you have completed the Walking 4 Wellness assessment, transfer your scores for each area of wellness (Body, Mind, Career & Finances, and Heart & Spirit) and compare your scores to the ideal "peak wellness" score for each area (see table below). Remember, don't beat yourself up—you'll probably find you are doing better in some areas and maybe not as well in others. That's OK. Our goal is to help you thrive in all four areas, but to do that we need to first identify your lowest scoring area. Next, create a "priority list" in the third column, based upon your lowest scores, ranking highest priority to the lowest scores. For example, let's imagine you scored 20 points for Body, 30 points for Mind, 25 points for Career & Finances, and Heart & Spirit = 15 points. Based upon these scores, your priority list would look like this: #1 Heart & Spirit, #2 Body, #3 Career & Finances, and #4 Mind.

Where to begin your journey? You are welcome to read the book in its entirety or, if you'd like, begin by reading your personal wellness priority areas first. You'll notice to the far right in the table below your Walking 4 Wellness Paths column. Here, specific chapters are listed with page numbers to help you begin your journey.

	PEAK WELLNESS SCORE	MY SCORE	MY PRIORITY	WALKING 4 WELLNESS PATHS
BODY	40			CHAPTER 2: Pages 30-49
MIND	40			CHAPTER 3: Pages 50-65
CAREER & FINANCES	40			CHAPTER 4: Pages 66-79
HEART & SPIRIT	40			CHAPTERS 5-6: Pages 80-103
TOTAL SCORE	160			CHAPTER 7: Pages 104-109

A Closer Look: What Your Score Means

Score of 35-40: If you scored between 35-40 points for a particular Walking 4 Wellness area, congratulations! Your answers indicate you are doing very well! You not only have an awareness of the importance of this area to your overall health and well-being—you also have developed the skills and habits to make this area so excellent! Well done! Keep up the great work in this area and you will reap the benefits of a healthy, fit and well balanced life. If for some reason you scored high in this area, but notice other areas struggling (e.g. Career/Finances are high but Body or Mind are low) be sure to devote time and energy to improving these other areas of your life while still maintaining the excellence you have created in this area.

Scores of 30-35: If you scored between 30-35 in one or more of your wellness areas, your health and wellness practices are considered good, but have room for improvement. Take a moment and identify all of the questions you may have scored yourself a 3 or lower and begin to think about subtle ways you can improve your score the next time you take this assessment.

Scores of 20-30: If you scored between 20-30 in one or more of your wellness areas, take a moment and identify all of the questions you may have scored yourself a 1 or a 2 and begin to consider your motivation, interest and confidence in improving these items. For example, you may have scored yourself a 1 or a 2 for "I maintain a healthy and desirable weight." This may be an ideal area to begin to focus your attention and set specific goals which you will find in the next step, "Plan Well."

Scores below 20: If you scored below a 20 in one or more of your Walking 4 Wellness areas it's time to begin to recapture your health and wellness. Look through these areas and identify what area you would most like to improve upon first. You can begin your journey wherever you would like, but you are much more apt to get started with the one you are most interested, motivated and confident you can change. Also, take a moment and identify all of the questions you may have scored yourself a 1 or a 2 and begin to assess your motivation and interests in improving this area. I would encourage you to begin to set specific goals to help you begin to make strides towards improving this area.

Assessing Your Health

Before you move on to planning your Walking 4 Wellness journey, take a moment to assess where you are today by answering a few additional questions and complete the suggested health and fitness tests.

Has your doctor ever said you have heart trouble?	YES	NO
Do you suffer frequent chest pains?	YES	NO
Do you often feel faint or have spells of severe dizziness?	YES	NO
Has your doctor ever told you that you have a bone or joint problem (arthritis) that has been aggravated or worsened by exercise?	YES	NO
Has your doctor ever said your blood pressure was too high?	YES	NO
Are you over age 65 and not accustomed to any exercise?	YES	NO
Are you taking any prescription medications, such as those for heart problems or high blood pressure?	YES	NO
Is there a good physical reason not mentioned here why you should not follow an activity program even if you wanted to?	YES	NO

If you answer "Yes" to any of these questions, I highly recommend consulting your physician before beginning your Walking 4 Wellness Program or any other exercise program.

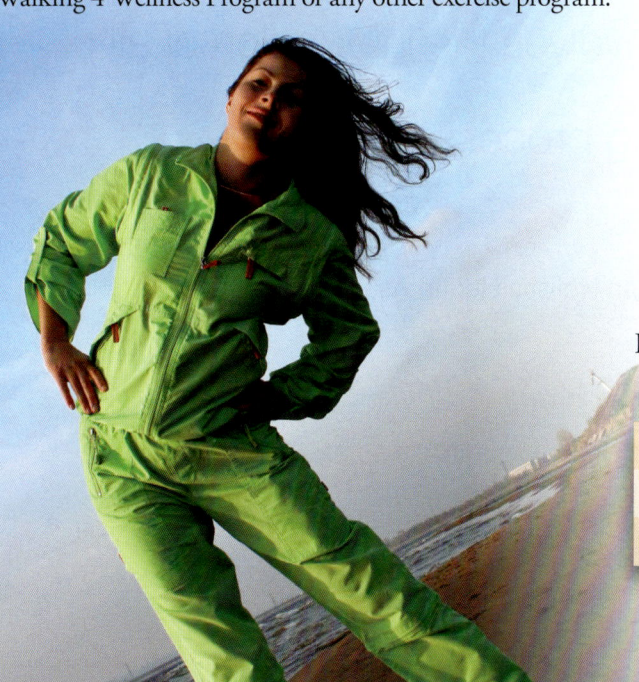

One Mile Walk Test

To evaluate your cardiovascular fitness as well as determine what Walking 4 Wellness style is best for you, take a moment to complete this simple test.

✓ **Goal**
  Walk a one-mile distance as fast as you can without jogging or running.

✓ **What You'll Need**
  1. A timer (smart phone or stopwatch) to monitor your time.

  2. A good pair of walking shoes.

  3. A designated one-mile walking area.

✓ **Instructions**
  1. Find a local high school track, walking trail or similar area where you can safely walk for a one-mile distance.

  2. Before you begin, be sure to warm up. (See page 37 for warm up instructions.)

  3. Once you have warmed up, begin your test by starting your timer.

  4. Walk as fast as you possibly can for the designated one-mile distance.

  5. Once you cover the one-mile distance stop the timer and record your score.

If you completed your one-mile walk in:

DURATION	STATUS
16 minutes or more	Novice/Beginner
13-15 minutes	Intermediate
12 minutes or less	Advanced

According to the World Health Organization, "Health is more than the absence of disease. Health is a state of optimal well-being." Optimal well-being is a concept of health that goes beyond the curing of illness to one of achieving wellness. Achieving wellness requires balancing the various aspects of the whole person. These aspects are physical, emotional, mental and spiritual. This broader, (w)holistic approach to health involves the integration of all of these aspects and is an ongoing process.

Wellness from Within: The First Step, The American Holistic Health Association

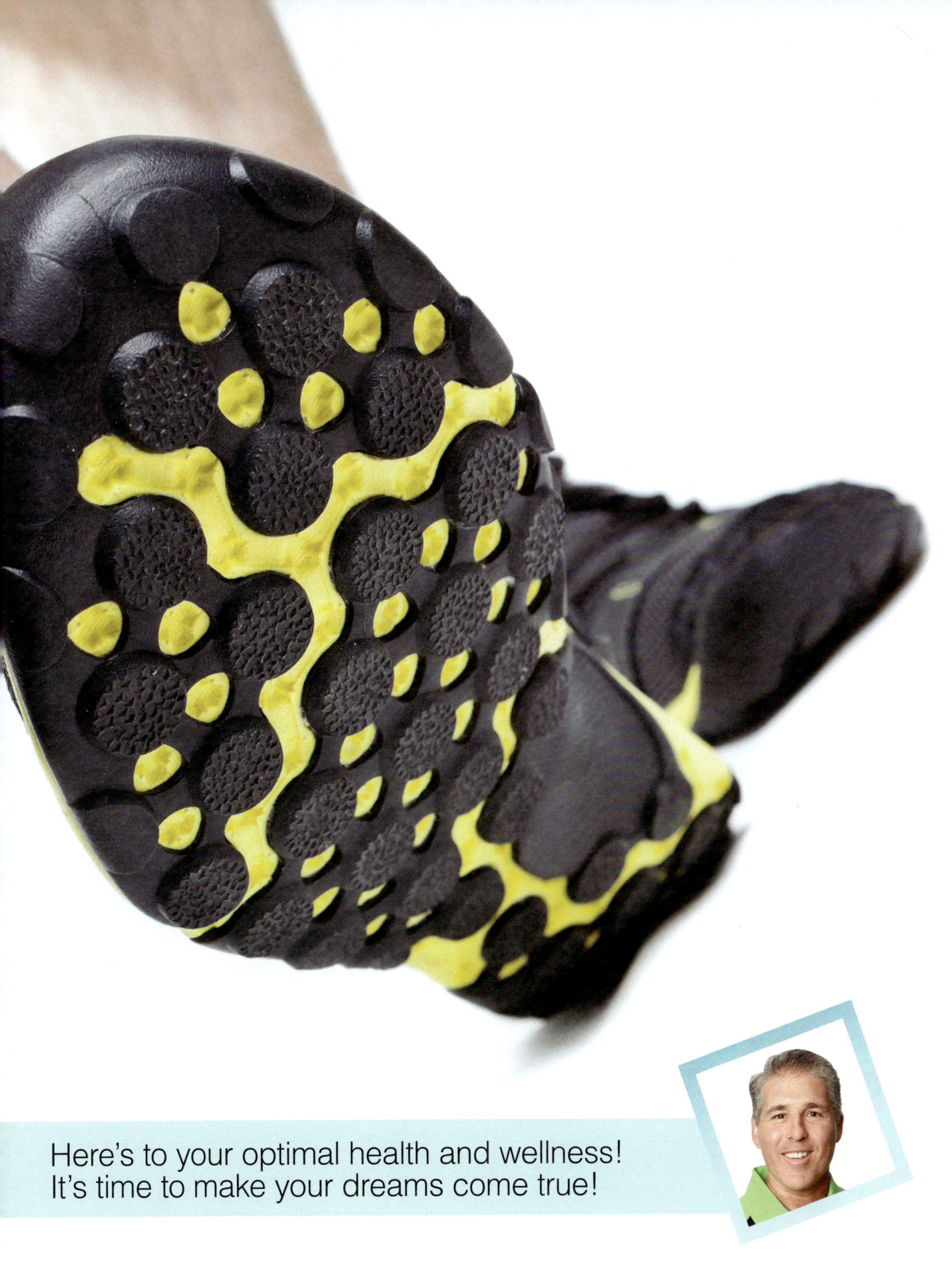

Here's to your optimal health and wellness!
It's time to make your dreams come true!

Four Simple Steps To Walk This Way

2 Plan Well: Casting Your Vision—Determining Your Destination

Setting your course to reach your desired destination of excellence in body, mind, career, heart and spirit can be compared in many respects to planning an expedition up a mountain or across a distant land. Anyone who has successfully reached their "peak" will tell you that it is essential to determine your final destination before you embark on your journey. Whether you are walking up a small hill or a mammoth mountain, whether you are a beginner or advanced status—all trips require proper planning,

training and appropriate resources to help you reach your desired "peak."

Now that you know where you are beginning, let's identify where you want to go. What's your destination? What's your "picture" or vision of your best body, emotional well-being, relationships, career and life? What does it look like? How does it feel? To help you begin to craft your Walking 4 Wellness vision, let's go back to our Wellness Mirror and your Walking 4 Wellness assessment you just took and ask yourself:

1 Related to my scores, if I continue to live the same way I am living today where do I see my body wellness 10 years from today?

☐ **Improving**   ☐ **Declining**   ☐ **Staying the same**

2 Related to my scores, if I continue to live the same way I am living today where do I see my mind wellness 10 years from today?

☐ **Improving**   ☐ **Declining**   ☐ **Staying the same**

3 Related to my scores, if I continue to live the same way I am living today where do I see my career and finance wellness 10 years from today?

☐ **Improving**   ☐ **Declining**   ☐ **Staying the same**

4 Related to my scores, if I continue to live the same way I am living today where do I see my heart and spirit wellness 10 years from today?

☐ **Improving**   ☐ **Declining**   ☐ **Staying the same**

5 Overall, how do I feel about my Walking 4 Wellness results?

☐ **Very Happy—I'm excelling in all four areas**

☐ **Mostly Satisfied—I'm excelling in at least three out of the four areas**

☐ **Concerned—I'm doing pretty well in at least two areas, but need to improve in the others**

☐ **Very Concerned—I need to make serious changes**

6 What's my "peak?" Ask yourself, "What would I like my health, wellness and life to look like 10 years from now? Picture yourself thriving physically, emotionally, financially and spiritually. What does this look like? How does it feel?

_____

_____

_____

7 To help make strides towards your "peak" you'll have the opportunity to begin your Walking 4 Wellness training over the coming weeks or months. To help you get started, set a distance and a goal of how far you would like to be able to walk one year from today:

- ☐ **5k Walk**
- ☐ **10k Walk**
- ☐ **½ Marathon**
- ☐ **Full Marathon**
- ☐ **Other** _____

8 Take a moment to identify the areas (at least one) of your personal wellness you would most like to improve. (Review your Walking 4 Wellness assessment priorities.) Write down your vision of what thriving in this specific area would look like as well as how long you plan to walk to commemorate your accomplishments—this will become your Walking 4 Wellness destination. For example, if my #1 priority is BODY and losing weight is one of my main interests, a personal vision or "peak" destination statement could be, "I will be 50 pounds lighter and walk a ½ marathon one year from today.")

- ☐ **Body** _____
- ☐ **Career & Finances** _____
- ☐ **Mind** _____
- ☐ **Heart & Spirit** _____

9 Select one statement that best describes your readiness to make the lifestyle change you selected above.

- ☐ **"I'm just not interested in working on changes in this area at the moment."**
- ☐ **"I'm thinking about improving this area of my life in the next few months."**
- ☐ **"I'm planning to begin to work on this area in the next month."**
- ☐ **"I am ready now to start working on this area of my life."**
- ☐ **"I have been actively working on improving my life in this area over at least the last six months."**

10 Determine a date when you would like to realize or reach your "peak" vision. _____
MONTH/DAY/YEAR

11 Sixteen weeks from now, what would you like to see, realize or accomplish to move you closer to your personal "peak" Walking 4 Wellness vision?

_____

12 Twelve weeks from now what would you like to see, realize or accomplish?

_____

13 Eight weeks from now what would you like to see, realize or accomplish?

_____

14 Four weeks from now what would you like to see, realize or accomplish?

_____

15 Rate your level of confidence in accomplishing your goals. (Circle the appropriate number for you—0 = No confidence, 5 = some confidence, 10 = total confidence.)

4 Week Goal	0	1	2	3	4	5	6	7	8	9	10
8 Week Goal	0	1	2	3	4	5	6	7	8	9	10
12 Week Goal	0	1	2	3	4	5	6	7	8	9	10
16 Week Goal	0	1	2	3	4	5	6	7	8	9	10
1 Year Goal	0	1	2	3	4	5	6	7	8	9	10
Peak Wellness Vision	0	1	2	3	4	5	6	7	8	9	10

Four Simple Steps To
Walk This Way

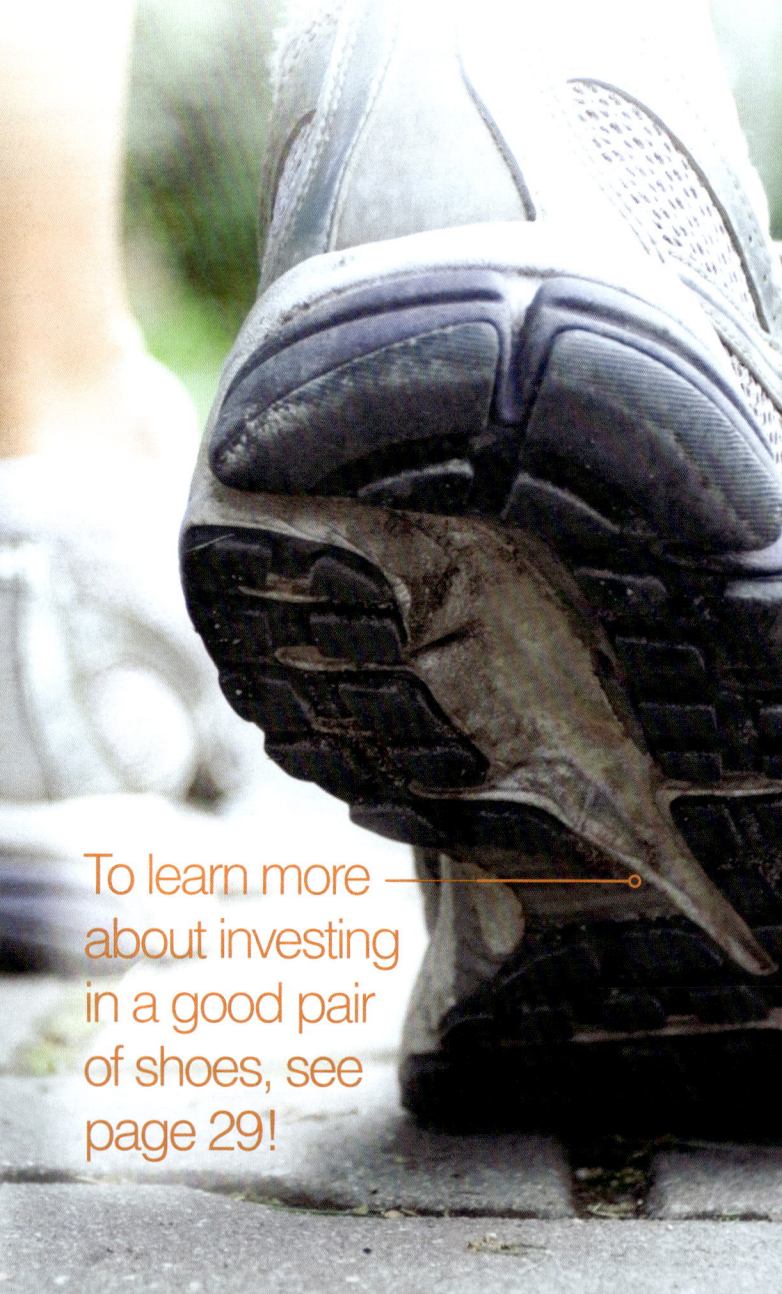

Four Walking Types

We've all heard of personality questionnaires, which tell us our "personality types," right? You know those fun inventories showing us our common personal traits, helping us understand what makes us tick. Well, did you know there are also different "Walking Types" that we all find ourselves gravitating towards based upon our goals, preferences and present fitness levels? Throughout this book you'll learn the best walking path for you and how to utilize different formats of walking to best reach your goals.

What's Your "Walking Type?"

To help you get started with your Walking 4 Wellness Plan, you'll want to take a moment to understand the four general types of walking you can consider. In the following chapters we will modify these walking styles with specific strategies to help you reach your desired goals. Take a moment to consider each walking type and see what fits you best:

1   **Strolling:** Casual walking

2   **Rolling:** Fast or power walking

3   **Burning:** Interval and terrain walking

4   **Toning:** Interval walking combined with resistance training

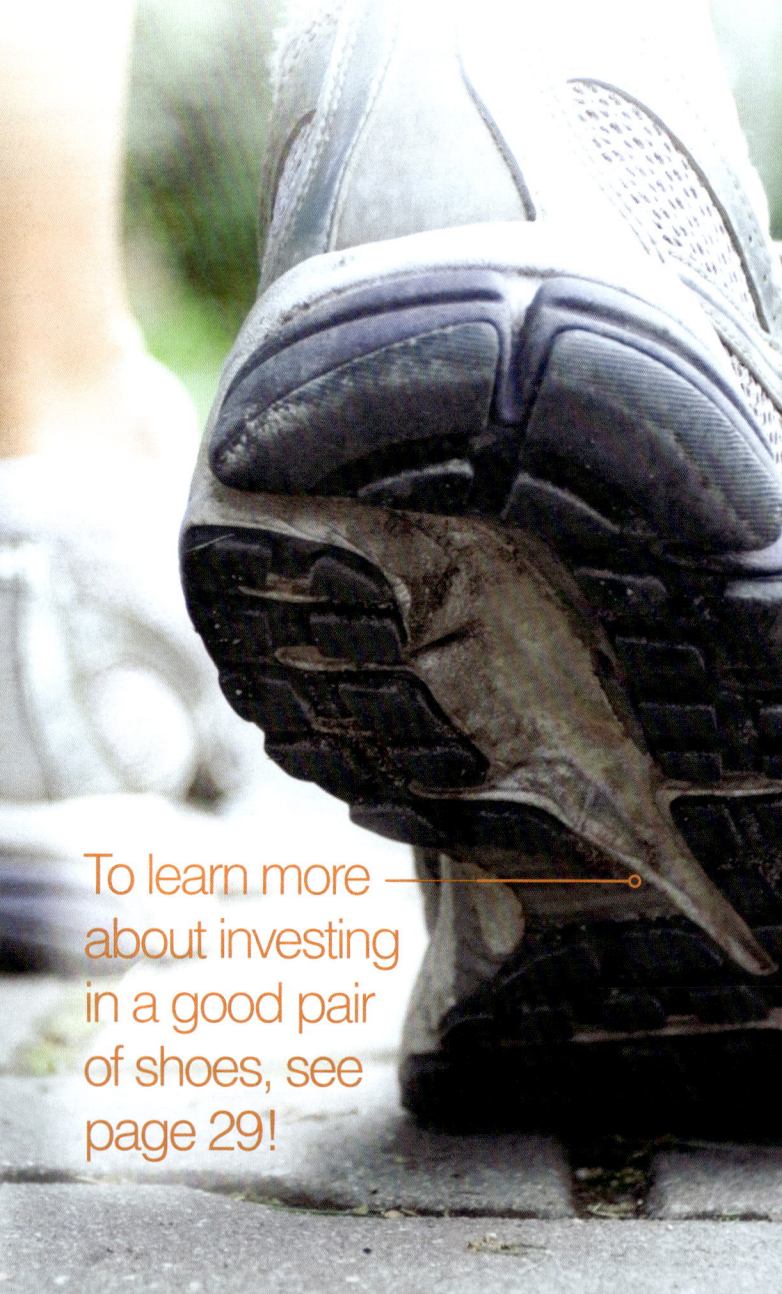
To learn more about investing in a good pair of shoes, see page 29!

1 Strolling Technique

If you find yourself enjoying a casual walk in the morning, middle or end of the day or if you resonate with a majority of the items listed below you may be best suited for "Strolling" or what is also known as "Recovery" walking. This type of walking is best for individuals who:

✓ Are beginners or are just getting back to walking or exercising

✓ Desire to improve their overall stamina, physical, emotional and spiritual health

✓ Enjoy tranquil, serene and meditative walks

✓ Are looking for a way to improve mood, decrease stress, relax and restore energy

✓ Prefer low intensity walking at a casual pace around 2.0-3.5 MPH

✓ Enjoy walking multiple times a day without perspiring too much

✓ Prefer slower, possibly longer walks

✓ Are interested in recovering from sore muscles or de-stressing

✓ Completed the One-Mile Walk Test in 16 minutes or more

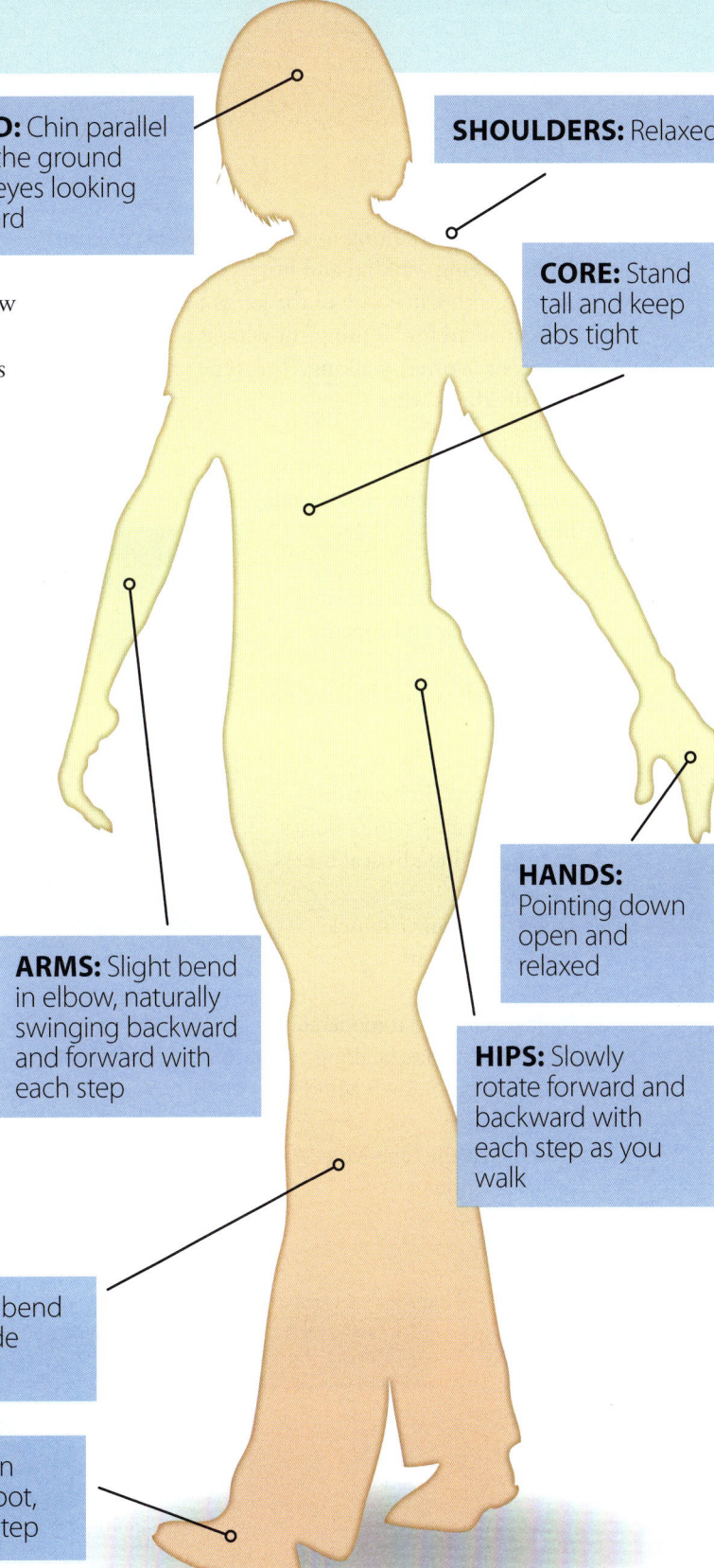

HEAD: Chin parallel with the ground with eyes looking forward

SHOULDERS: Relaxed

CORE: Stand tall and keep abs tight

HANDS: Pointing down open and relaxed

ARMS: Slight bend in elbow, naturally swinging backward and forward with each step

HIPS: Slowly rotate forward and backward with each step as you walk

LEGS: Slight bend in knees, stride comfortably

FEET: Lead with the heel, touch down briefly and transfer weight to ball of foot, push from ball of the foot with each step

Four Simple Steps To
Walk This Way

2 Rolling Technique

If you find yourself wanting to step it up and experience a more challenging walking and fitness regimen or if you resonate with a majority of the items below you may be best suited for "Rolling" or what is also known as "Fitness" or "Power" walking. This type of walking is best for individuals who:

✓ Desire to improve productivity, creativity, resilience and overall fitness

✓ Are interested in decreasing stress, anxiety and appetite

✓ Enjoy moderate to challenging exercise

✓ Are interested in increasing energy, burning more calories and improving physical fitness

✓ Desire to enhance muscle and bone strength

✓ Prefer exercising at moderate to higher intensities, walking at a pace ranging from 3.5-4.5 MPH

✓ Completed the One-Mile Walk Test in 13-15 minutes

HEAD: Ears in alignment with shoulders with chin level to the ground

CHEST: Slightly lifted

SHOULDERS: Down and relaxed

CORE: Stand tall, lean forward slightly from ankles

ARMS: Bend at 90 degrees, close to your hips and swing forward and back

HANDS: Loosely cupped with index finger and thumb touching

HIPS: Under shoulders, rotating forward and backward as you walk

LEGS: With slight bend in knees, take natural fast steady strides

FEET: Draw toes to shin, place heel to the ground, "roll" the foot propelling forward from toes

3 Burning Technique

If you find yourself wanting to take your walking to another level and burn more body fat or if you resonate with a majority of the items below you may be best suited for "Burning" or what is also known as "Interval" training. This type of walking is best for individuals who:

✓ Desire to maximize fat burning and weight loss

✓ Are interested in shorter, more challenging workouts

✓ Desire to boost energy, mood and reduce belly fat

✓ Are interested in toning, strengthening and defining muscles

✓ Prefer varying walking/running speed from moderate to fast, ranging intensities from 4.5-6.5 MPH

✓ Enjoy using different speeds, terrains or elevations to impact intensity

✓ Completed the One-Mile Walk Test in under 13 minutes

HEAD: Eyes straight ahead chin level to ground

SHOULDERS: Down and relaxed, don't allow to raise up to ears

CHEST: Slightly elevated

HANDS: Loosely cupped

ARMS: Elbows close to torso, bent at 90 degrees

CORE: Abs tight, pull belly into spine with slight natural lean

HIPS: Under shoulders, rotating forward and backward, not side to side

FEET: Strike the mid-foot under center of gravity with toes pointing downward, lightly land on ball and push ground away from you

Four Simple Steps To Walk This Way

4 Toning Technique

If you find yourself wanting to take a bigger jump in your wellness, fitness and health and move up to the next level of walking or if you resonate with a majority of the items below you may be best suited for "Toning" or what is also known as "Circuit Walking." This type of walking combines walking along with resistance oriented exercises using body weight or equipment in a circuit fashion. This type of walking is best for individuals who:

✓ Are interested in slowing the aging process and looking and feeling years younger

✓ Desire to shape, strengthen and define upper and lower body muscles

✓ Would like to maximize metabolism and fat burning ability throughout the day

✓ Want to get fit and stay fit

✓ Prefer utilizing fitness tools, resistance equipment or body weight exercises along with their walking

✓ Vary walking/running speeds ranging from 4.5-6.5 MPH along with resistance training

✓ Completed the One-Mile Walk Test in under 13 minutes

You'll use the same walking technique as "Burning" alternating your speeds between moderate and fast paced walking/running, but now will add a little twist. Now you'll be adding toning exercises using your body weight or portable resistance equipment throughout your walk. This is a great way to reverse the aging process and get fit fast.

Congratulations! You are one step closer to realizing your dream. Now please turn to your selected Walking 4 Wellness path or the next chapter:

Chapter 2: Body

Chapter 3: Mind

Chapter 4: Career & Finances

Chapter 5 & 6: Heart & Spirit

Chapter 7: Creating Your Plan

Rise & Shine!

Starting your morning with a healthy walk can make for a more productive day!

Important Note: Invest In A Good Pair Of Shoes!

Wearing the right shoes will make Walking 4 Wellness a pleasure and not a pain and save you from potential blisters, calluses and injuries. Think about the steps below when purchasing your walking shoes:

- Consider shopping at a shoe specialty store to have your shoes fitted for you, to protect your feet and your body. A little extra investment is well worth it.

- If you're already an experienced walker, bring an old pair of shoes with you to the store and show them to the salesperson—it's additional evidence to help determine how you normally walk. By looking at your shoes you can determine if you have a low, high or neutral arch. According to Duke University, if you have normal wear and tear across your shoe, you most likely have a neutral arch (you'll want to look for "Stability Shoes"—extra arch side support and high density foam). If you have a low arch, the inner soles of your shoe will be worn (you'll want to look for "Motion control shoes" which have increased stability and filled in arches). If you have a high arch, the outer soles of your shoe will be excessively worn (you'll want to look for "Cushioning Shoes" light weight, flexible with minimal rigidity and extra cushioning).

- Go shopping at the end of the day, as our feet tend to swell, and be sure to wear the same type of sock you'll be walking in.

- Be sure to have both feet measured, as one foot is usually larger than the other.

- Don't forget to stand when measuring your feet.

- When sizing your shoes, make sure you can wiggle your toes. There should be a half inch distance between your longest toe and the end of the shoe.

- Also, check the width and also the heel—they should feel snug, but not tight.

- Walk around the store before buying your shoes and ask about their return policy. Many stores will allow you to walk for a week or so and if they don't fit well, most reputable stores will take them back.

- Be sure to check your foot size every year. Your feet actually may grow as you get older.

- Replace your shoes on a regular basis. Most experts agree, for every 500 miles it's time for a new pair of shoes. Remember, with each step and mile you are breaking down the cushion of the shoe. General rule: If you walk for an hour or so three times a week you should be replacing your shoes every five to six months.

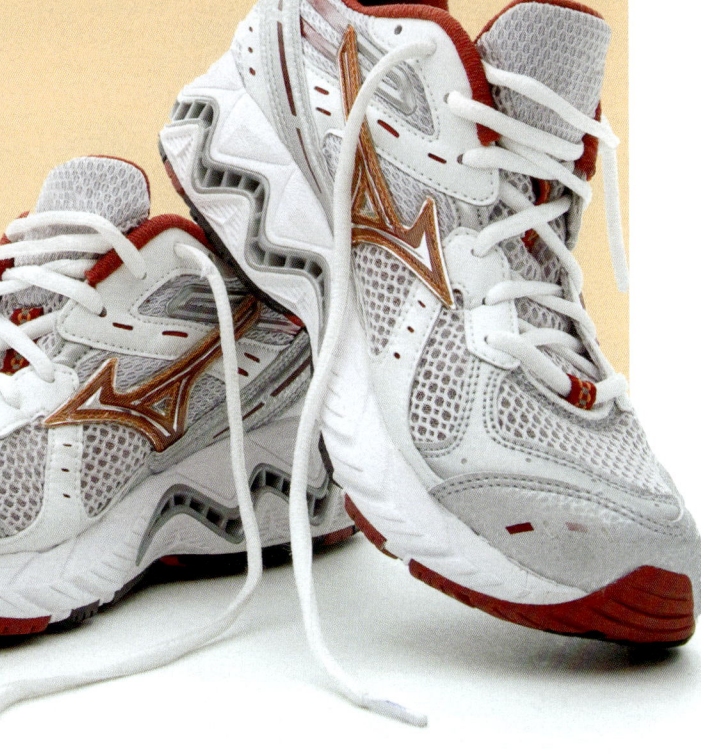

Chapter 2

Walking 4 Your Body

Simple Steps To Lose Weight, Get Fit & Experience Optimal Health!

Success will never be a big step in the future;
Success is a small step taken just now.

JONATAN MARTENSSON

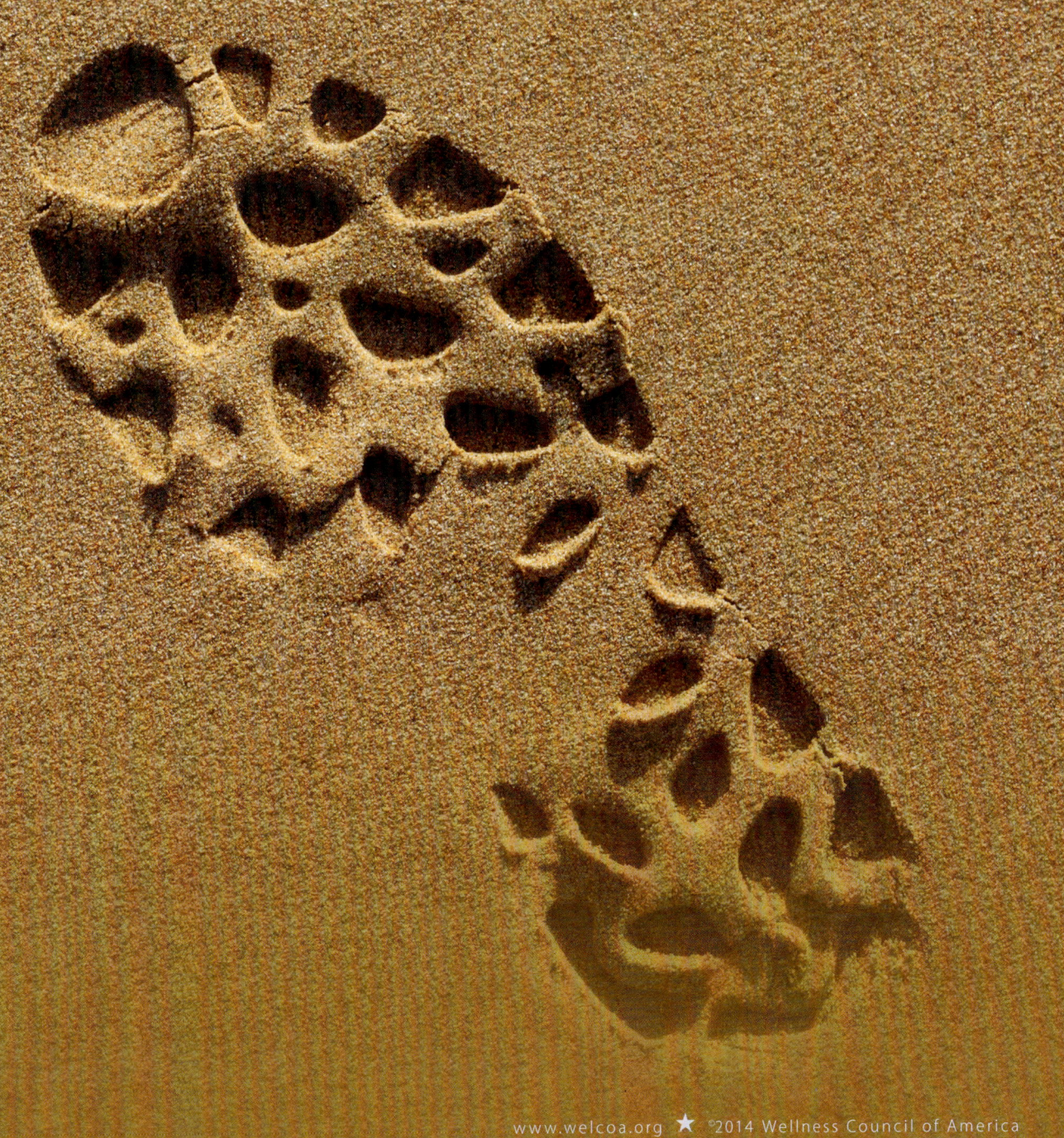

Walking 4 Your Body

Sleepless To Shapely

It's 2:00 AM and Dana can't sleep again. With busy thoughts racing in and out of her head, she walks down stairs to the kitchen, first grabbing a snack and then, like clock work, on to the living room where she picks up the TV remote to watch hours of infomercials. Sadly, over the last year and a half, this erratic sleep schedule has become a regular ritual along with endless purchases of the latest "Miracle Diet" books, "Fitness DVD systems," or "Breakthrough Slimming Pills." Like a driven scientist seeking a cure for the common cold, Dana scours the TV airwaves, desperately hunting for a solution for her nagging insomnia, high blood pressure and especially the stubborn extra 50 pounds she can't seem to get off her body or out of her head.

One night, Dana stumbles upon a talk show discussing the power of walking and weight loss. She quickly changes the channel as she reminds herself of the hefty purchase she made of "the latest and greatest exercise program" six months ago, which left her in bed for three days with a sore back and no weight loss. But for some reason, Dana turned back to the program and began to listen to the panel of experts along with stories of amazing health, fitness and weight loss success. "Thirty pounds." "Eighty pounds." "One hundred and fifty pounds," all gone! "Lower blood pressure." "More energy." "Improved sleep." One after the other, each individual sharing how they finally got fed up with all the gimmicks and decided to put one foot in front of the other and begin a different journey to realize their goals by simply walking. Next, a panel of medical experts shared the many health and fitness benefits of walking as well as an easy-to-follow approach anyone could use to help boost their metabolism and burn up to nine times more body fat. Dana was intrigued and inspired by their stories, the research and the price—it was free! The next day she decided to take the advice of those who were on the show and began to walk that evening. Since that night Dana has never purchased another infomercial gadget

or gimmick again. She is now proudly 50 pounds lighter and has been walking ever since. Not only has she reached her dream weight, feeling healthier, younger, more energetic, fitter and happier than she's ever been in years, she also says the best part is, "I can fit in clothes I only dreamed I'd be able to wear again and I can actually sleep through the night! But my husband would tell you, beyond losing all the weight and looking like I did 20 years ago, the best part is we've saved a ton of money!"

Can you relate to Dana? Maybe you are struggling with low energy or lack of sleep or rising blood pressure or stubborn extra weight? You may be searching, like Dana, for a real solution to address all of your health and fitness concerns. What if I were to tell you there is such a "cure" and it can be discovered by following a proven path? We call it Walking 4 Your Body.

In this chapter, you'll discover exactly how to boost your body's ability to lose weight, and you'll experience dramatic changes to your health and fitness, and much, much more. We will explore:

1 **Why Walk:** Anatomy of Walking 4 Your Body

2 **Getting Started:** Answering Your Body Questions

3 **Plan Well:** How To Warm Your Body Up

4 **Walk 4 Weight Loss:** Proven strategies and tips to help you lose weight and keep it off

5 **How To Lose Nine Times More Body Fat:** Your 4-Week Walking 4 Your Body Workouts

After reading this chapter you'll have the map to make your health, fitness and body dreams a reality.

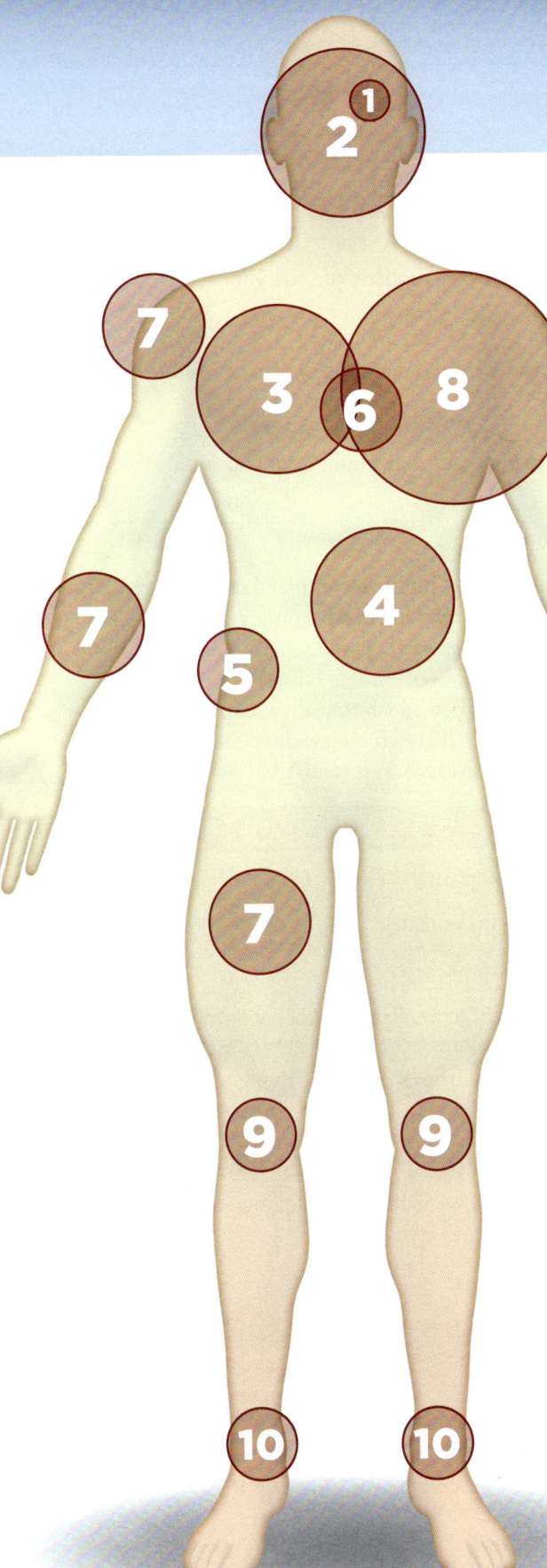

Why Walk: Anatomy Of Walking 4 Your Body

Researchers from the American College of Sports Medicine, the American Heart Association, Harvard University, the Mayo Clinic and a host of additional national and international organizations all agree that walking is one of the best things you can do for your body. Overwhelming scientific evidence supports the growing number of positive benefits for your body and health by putting one foot in front of the other. Take a look at just a few of the many benefits your body will experience by walking on a regular basis, such as:

❶ **Improves eye health—reducing risk of glaucoma.**

❷ **Keeps skin young and supple—look and feel years younger.**

❸ **Improves lung capacity.**

❹ **Manage your body weight, improve metabolism and increase your ability to burn fat.**

❺ **Strengthen bones.**

❻ **Increases energy, reduces blood pressure, increases "good" cholesterol and lowers your risk of heart disease.**

❼ **Strengthen and improve tone of core, legs, shoulders and arms.**

❽ **Reduces risk of cancer.**

❾ **Helps with arthritis—relieves stiffness and improves range of motion in joints.**

❿ **Improve balance and coordination.**

Plus: Lowers risk of diabetes and strengthens immune system.

Walking 4 Your Body

Getting Started

Before you begin your Walking 4 Wellness Plan follow the steps below to properly prepare yourself:

Ask The Right Body Questions:

To help you Walk 4 Your Body and track your personal progress, take a moment to complete the following questions and optional body tests:

1 Do you have any physical limitations (injury, joint discomfort, etc.) that would limit you from participating in a regular walking program?

☐ Yes   ☐ No

If you answered yes, before beginning this or any other fitness program, I highly recommend consulting a physician or health professional to receive appropriate instruction in following a safe and effective program for you.

Assessing Your Activity Throughout Your Day:

2 During your typical workday (for example, from 9 AM to 5 PM) how much time do you spend sitting? (You can assess the number of hours you sit by keeping a "sitting diary" for a few days. Simply add the total number of hours you sit over a three-day period and then average your totals).

✓	Typically, how much do you sit during your work day?
	I sit 6 or more hours, at a time, with no physical movement during my work day.
	I sit 4-5 hours, at a time, with some light movements during my work day.
	I sit 2-3 hours, at a time, with moderate movements during my work day.
	I sit less than 1-2 hours, at a time, along with participating in very active/physical labor during my work day.

3 How many hours a day would you estimate you are sitting away from work (e.g. driving to and from work, leisure time at home, watching TV)?

My total number of hours sitting down, away from work is: _____

4 Do you regularly, within the last month, perform aerobic activities such as walking, jogging or cycling at least four times per week for 20-60 minutes?

☐ Yes   ☐ No   ☐ Sometimes

5 How would you rate your cardiovascular endurance?

☐ Excellent   ☐ Good   ☐ Average   ☐ Needs Attention

6 Do you regularly, within the last month, perform strength training exercises such as push-ups or squats or sit-ups using either your body weight, free weights, dumbbells or resistance bands, at least two-three times per week?

☐ Yes   ☐ No   ☐ Sometimes

7 How would you rate your current upper body strength?
☐ Excellent ☐ Good ☐ Average ☐ Needs Attention

8 How would you rate your current lower body strength?
☐ Excellent ☐ Good ☐ Average ☐ Needs Attention

9 How would you rate your abdominal strength?
☐ Excellent ☐ Good ☐ Average ☐ Needs Attention

10 Do you regularly, within the last month, perform stretching exercises for the upper and lower body, such as overhead arm stretches, hamstring, calf or quadriceps stretches at least four times per week?
☐ Yes ☐ No

11 Would you rate your flexibility as good to excellent?
☐ Yes ☐ No

12 How would you rate your current body composition?
☐ Excellent ☐ Good ☐ Average ☐ Needs Attention

13 How would you rate your overall fitness?
☐ Excellent ☐ Good ☐ Average ☐ Needs Attention

I'd recommend re-testing yourself every four to six weeks for the tests you are most interested in measuring Walking 4 Your Body progress.

Walking 4 Your Body

Recommended Walking 4 Your Body Tracking:

To help you further track your body progress consider completing the following:

1 Track your weight:

Body Weight	Week 1	Week 4	Week 8	Week 12	Week 16

2 Take a before and after picture of yourself.

3 Track your "energy level" on a scale of 0-10 over a three-day period, using this journal or a smart phone.

Energy Level (0 = None, 5 = Some, 10 = Boundless)	Day 1	Day 2	Day 3

4 Monitor health-related information (e.g. blood pressure, blood cholesterol, body composition, bone density or lung function)

5 Measure yourself:

Body Measurements	Week 1	Week 4	Week 8	Week 12	Week 16
Arms					
Waist					
Hips					
Thighs					

6 Perform optional additional fitness tests:

a. Push-up test—Perform as many as you can: _____

b. Pull-up test—Perform as many as you can: _____

c. Sit-up or curl-up test—Perform as many as you can in one minute: _____

d. Measure your flexibility (Touch toes, measure distance away from or overlapping your toes): _____

e. One mile walk test—walk one mile as fast as you can (See page 19 for instructions): _____

I'd recommend re-testing yourself every 4-6 weeks for the tests you are most interested in measuring Walking 4 Your Body progress.

Plan Well: Always Warm Up

Be sure you always warm up your body by walking at a comfortable "strolling pace" for at least three to five minutes as well as adding upper and lower body movements (see below) to get the kinks out:

1 **Heel Raises.** Place your feet hip width apart. Next, raise up on the balls of your feet as high as you can, tighten calves, hold for two seconds, then lower down. Repeat 10-15 times.

2 **Toe Taps.** Place your right foot slightly in front of your left. Next, tap your right foot, raising toes up towards your shin and down. Repeat 20 times each leg.

3 **Ankle Circles.** Stand on your left leg/foot with right foot extended in front of you. Next, make a circular motion with your right foot 10 times in each direction. Repeat with the other foot.

4 **Forward And Backward Leg Swings.** While standing on your left leg/foot, raise your right leg, from the hip, in front of you (as if you were kicking someone in front of you) and then gently swing your leg behind you (as if you were kicking someone behind you). Perform this motion 10 times on each leg.

5 **Side-To-Side Leg Swings.** Just like the forward and backward leg swing, but this time swing your leg out to the side, away from the midline of your body and then back across your body. While standing on your left leg, raise your right leg out to the side, from the hip, and then gently swing your leg across your body. Repeat motion and perform 10 times on each leg.

6 **Shoulder Circles.** Stand with your feet shoulder width apart, knees slightly bent and your arms extended out to your sides, raised to shoulder level and palms facing the floor. Next, begin to make small forward circular motions (about one foot in diameter) with your hands and arms in a controlled and slow fashion. Then begin to slowly increase the size of your shoulder arm circles by progressing to medium to larger circular motions, until you are reaching as far forward and back as you comfortably can (e.g. above your head and below your hips). Perform 10 times forward and 10 times backwards (reversing the motion).

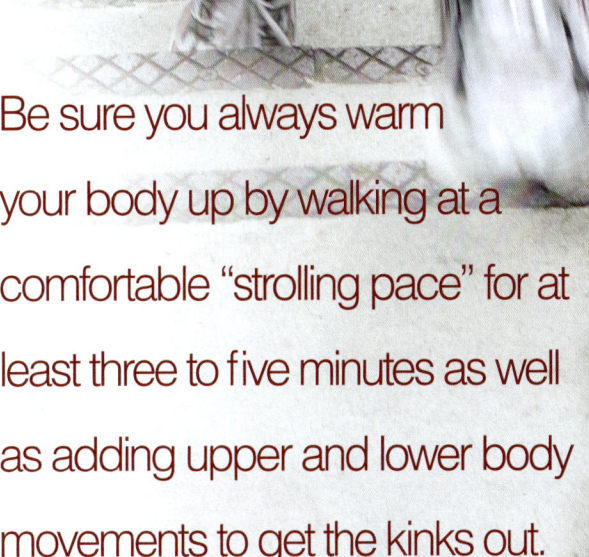

Be sure you always warm your body up by walking at a comfortable "strolling pace" for at least three to five minutes as well as adding upper and lower body movements to get the kinks out.

Walking 4 Your Body

Walk Well: Walking 4 Weight Loss

As mentioned, walking can significantly improve your health and fitness. But did you know that adding just a few nutritional strategies along with a regular walking program will dramatically impact your ability to lose weight and manage it for good? According to the prestigious National Weight Control Registry analysis of over 4,200 individuals, there are four common strategies discovered among successful "losers" consistently used to not only lose weight but also to keep it off:

1 EAT MORE TO LOSE WEIGHT! Researchers are making it clear, eating five to nine servings or more of vegetables and fruits a day not only improves your health and energy, it can also help you lose weight. Registry researchers identified the majority of individuals who ate more vegetables, fruits, whole grains and lean protein (a higher complex carbohydrates and lower fat diet) consistently lost and stayed at their desired weight. Many additional researchers have concluded that eating an abundance of these high fiber foods may be one of the most effective strategies to not only reducing disease but also helping manage weight "naturally." According to the Mayo Clinic, eating more of a variety of lower calorie plant-based foods, such as vegetables and fruits aids in suppressing appetite and naturally helps you feel satisfied throughout your day. To avoid deprivation and the old diet mentality you may want to think first about

what you can add to your daily diet verses what you need to take away. Here are some simple tips to help you:

A Keep track of how many fruits and vegetables you eat daily. You are much more likely to eat more veggies and fruits if you see how many servings you are getting written down in "black and white."

B Lose weight with color. Start your lunch or dinner with a salad loaded with all the colors of the rainbow (for example, red = tomatoes; green = romaine lettuce, broccoli; purple = eggplant; white = mushrooms; and yellow = squash) or a color-filled vegetable soup.

C Fill half of your dinner plate with an array of colorful vegetables.

D Add berries to your breakfast. Add an array of berries to your cereal (for example; blueberries, blackberries, strawberries or cranberries).

E Dip 'em. For healthy snacks, cut up carrots, tomatoes, cucumbers and celery and dip in plain yogurt with salsa.

F Load up. When going to the store load up on fruits and veggies and then make sure they're readily available at home (e.g. fruit bowl, cut veggies in containers easily seen in refrigerator).

G Enjoy "Fast Food." Re-frame the way you think of "fast food." When on the go, grab an apple, pear, plum or banana for a healthy snack.

*National Registry researchers also identified individuals lost weight on a number of different diet plans such as high protein and low carbohydrate but discovered those who kept it off the best were those who followed the complex carbohydrate approach.

Want Some More **Walking 4 Weight Loss** Tips?

1. **Drink up—water that is!** By consuming an abundance of water throughout your day, not only will you naturally suppress your appetite, but you'll also do one of the best things for your digestion, metabolism, skin and body as well as minimize any additional calories from other beverages. Here are a couple of tips to help you get your water in:

   - Try drinking ½ your body weight in ounces.

   - Use your smart phone alarm to remind you every hour to drink a glass of water at work (e.g. eight hours = eight glasses of water).

   - Keep a water bottle with you at all times. Take regular sips throughout the day.

   - Before eating a snack or meal prep your pallet with a large glass of water.

   - Track your water intake on your smart phone or a journal throughout the day.

   - Flavor your water with lemon or lime.

2. **Watch your speed.** Slowing the pace at which you eat will not only reduce your food intake, but it will also increase your enjoyment of food. By taking the time to savor the taste of your food and appreciate its aroma, texture and appearance, you make the process of eating much more mindful and satisfying. Below you will find some additional tips to help you learn how to slow your eating speed!

   - Identify how fast you eat; set a timer for two minutes and count how long it takes you in between bites during that period of time.

   - Minimize your distractions. Turn the TV off. Also, pay attention to what you are eating, where you are sitting or standing and the taste and texture of your food.

   - Practice deep breathing in between bites.

   - Put your fork down in between bites.

   - Drink water or use a napkin in between bites.

   - Eat with your opposite hand.

   - Enjoy conversation while eating.

   - Cut food into smaller portions.

3. **Avoid late night eating.** Avoid eating three hours before going to bed. Here are a few ideas to help:

   - Consider drinking herbal tea with mint or chamomile to replace dessert.

   - Brush your teeth right after your dinner.

   - Adopt the motto "anything after eight is too late."

4. **Control your portions.** According to best selling author and nutritional expert, Dr. Ann Kulze, MD, controlling your appetite and portions may be one of the biggest challenges when it comes to managing weight. Here are a few of her tried and true suggestions to help manage your portions:

   - When dining out, request that your server package half of your meal in a take-home box before you are served.

   - Have an appetizer as your main dish.

   - Split an entrée with your dining partner.

   - Request a smaller portion.

   - Avoid large buffet lines and all-you-can-eat restaurants. Studies show the more quantity and variety available to us, the more we eat.

   - Also, you may want to consider using smaller plates and bowls. Using smaller versions of your serving items may help you eat less food without even thinking about it. For more proven nutritional strategies from Dr. Ann, check out her latest book, *"Weigh Less for Life."*

5. **Out of sight out of mind.** Keep healthier food items in your home in plain sight for you and your family to see. If you are up to it, clean out your pantry and refrigerator and get rid of all foods that trigger and tempt you. Or, take small steps and put tempting foods in plastic, opaque containers in a designated area or drawer.

6. **Remember, you don't have to be perfect to be healthy and fit.** Being fit and healthy does not mean you have to be perfect. When you overeat or have the occasional snack at night, don't beat yourself up, identify what triggered your appetite, learn from it and recommit to your goal, and get back on track the next day!

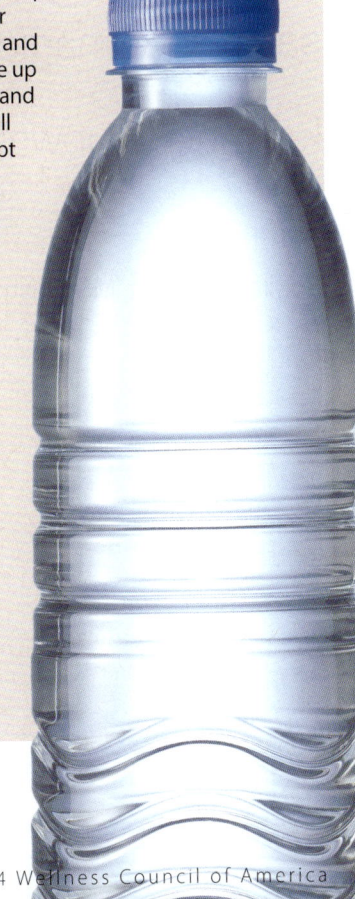

The Magic Pill

"I would say committing to physical activity, to a physical lifestyle, is the single most important thing people can do to prevent the buildup of belly fat and get rid of existing belly fat. Moderate-intensity physical activity (like walking), I would say is the "magic pill" because the health benefits go beyond keeping your waistline trim!"

Sheila A. Dugan, MD Rush University Medical Center

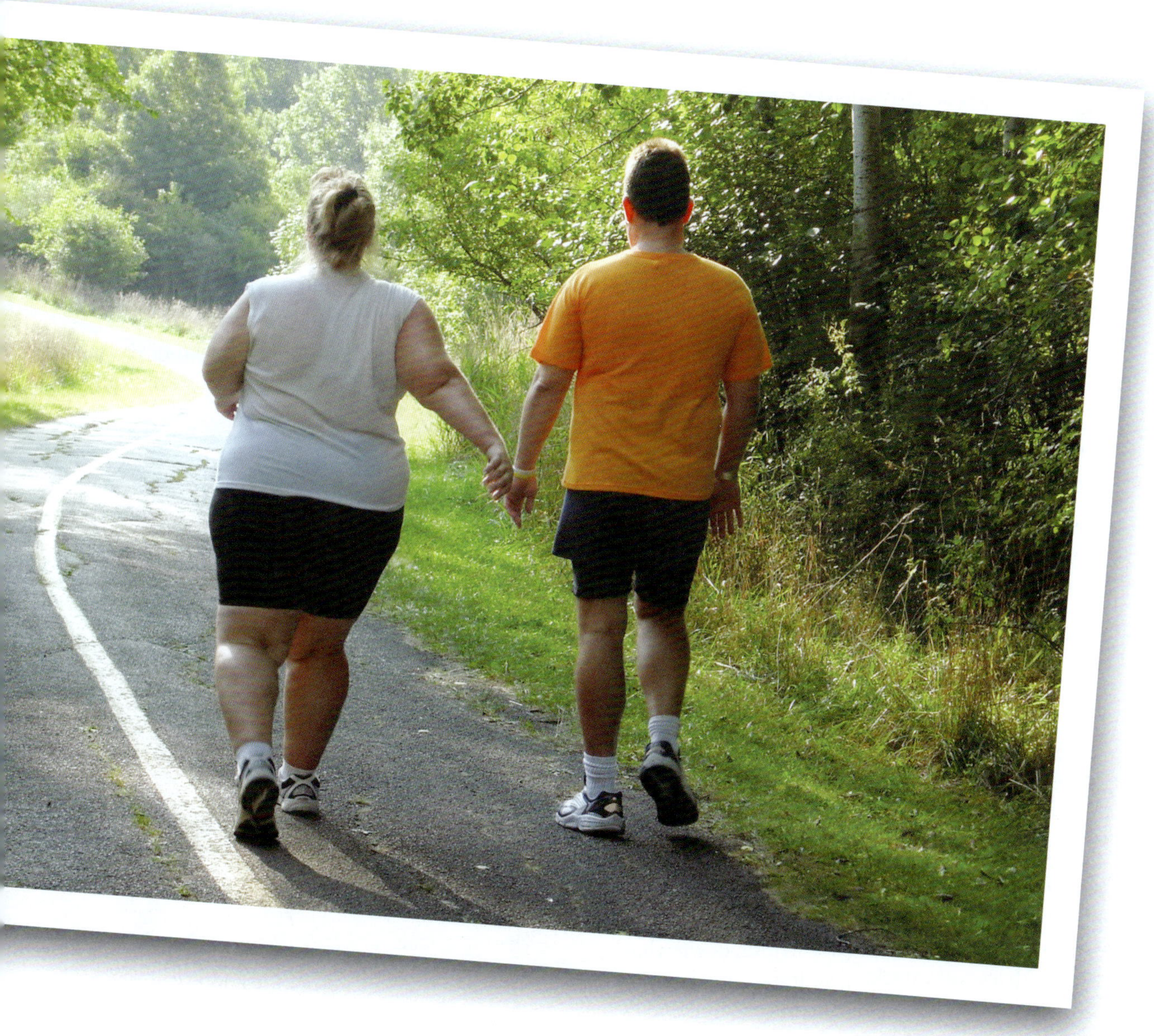

I always tell my clients, "The best exercise to help you lose weight or get in shape is the one you will do! Consistency is the key to success."

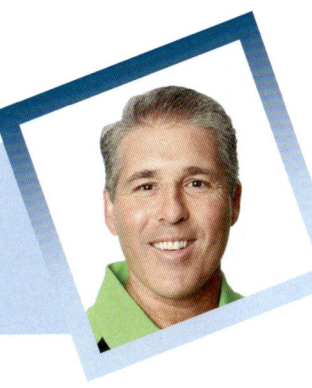

Walking 4 Your Body

2 START YOUR DAY RIGHT: EAT BREAKFAST!

Registry researchers also identified successful "losers", those who maintained their weight loss for over three years, were those who also consistently ate a healthy breakfast. With over 78% of "successful losers" reporting eating breakfast, researchers postulate eating a healthy meal may set the tone for the rest of your day as the majority of breakfast eaters were also more active. To help you eat a consistent healthy breakfast think about:

A Planning ahead. Determine what you will have for breakfast the night before and prep items for the next morning.

B Breakfast on the go. Enjoy a handful of walnuts and a cup of Greek yogurt or a glass of almond milk with frozen strawberries and protein powder for a quick nutritious smoothie.

C Combine three different foods for breakfast. A quick, energy starting carbohydrate (fruit), a long lasting whole grain complex carbohydrate (whole grain cereals), and a power building protein (dairy, egg, soy, meat or whey protein powder).

3 TRACK YOUR WEIGHT, ACTIVITY AND FOOD.

Registry researchers have identified a regular weekly weigh-in significantly aids with weight loss as well as weight maintenance. Also writing down what you eat on a daily basis, tracking your daily food intake, physical activity and other items such as cravings and emotions has been identified as one of the best strategies to not only help you lose weight but also keep it off.

4 MOVE EVERY DAY: SURPRISE, SURPRISE!

With over 94% of "successful losers" performing physical activity and exercise, Registry researchers identified walking to be the most popular form of exercise amongst its massive database. Researchers have also discovered individuals perform different types of walking to meet their desired goals and interests, all contributing to a healthier, happier lifestyle.

Walk Well: Lacing Up Your Shoes

Now that you've learned some proven nutritional strategies to help with walking and weight loss, you are ready to select the walking path that will work best for you. In the following pages you'll find four different four-week walking workouts you can select from and advance yourself to. If you'd like a refresher on what type of walking is best for you, go to pages 24 to 28. Be sure and select the type of walking workout you feel most confident you can accomplish and are physically ready to perform.

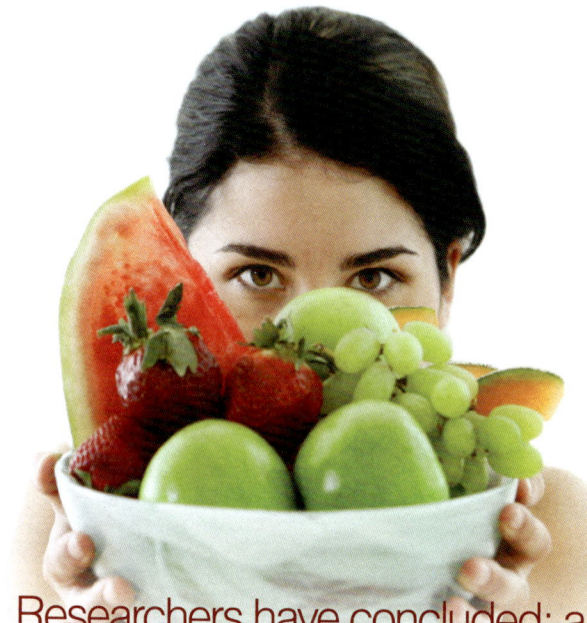

Researchers have concluded; a healthy balanced diet combined with regular exercise, such as walking seems to be the magic potion to help successful "losers" to not only lose weight but also keep it off.

www.welcoa.org

Walking 4 Your Body Workout #1: "Strolling"

Goal—Accumulate at least 30 minutes of physical activity most days of the week:

✓ To boost your energy and combat "sitting disease", strolling is one of the best ways to get going during your day. When seated at your desk, get up, walk or "march" in place for one to two minutes every hour.

✓ "Stroll" to the copy machine or get a drink of water every hour.

✓ Take your colleagues for a 10 minute or longer "walk-n-talk" meeting by strolling around the office building.

✓ Park your car further away and stroll into work.

✓ Stroll up the stairs instead of using the elevator.

✓ Stroll for 10 minutes in the morning, at lunch and after dinner.

✓ On a scale of 1-10, 1 = Easy, light breathing, 5 = Somewhat winded, and 10 = Racing someone full speed, almost breathless; perform "Strolling" at a 2-5 intensity level.

"Strolling" Walking For Your Body Workout—Week 1 Goal: Four days per week.

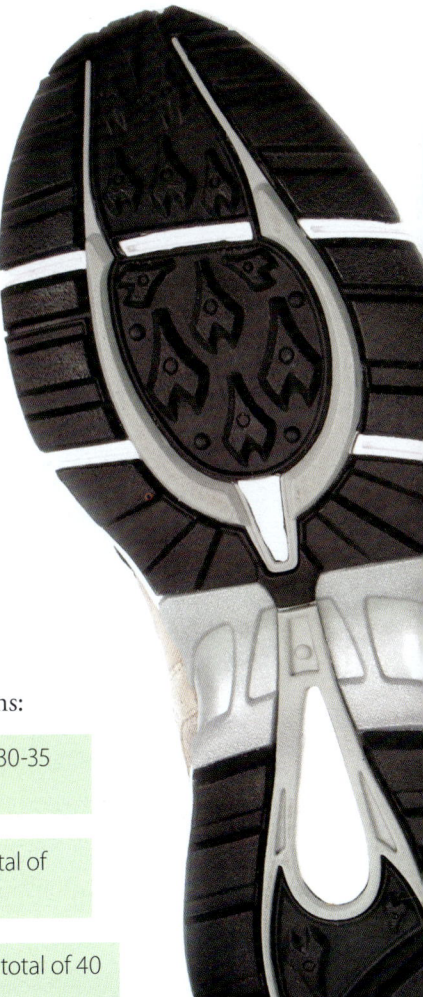

☼ DAY	🕐 WALKING WORKOUT	☰ INTENSITY
Monday	Strolling-Walk 10 minutes 3× a day or 30 minutes a day	2-3
Tuesday	Strolling-Walk 10 minutes 3× a day or 30 minutes a day	2-3
Wednesday	Rest	
Thursday	Strolling-Walk 10 minutes 3× a day or 30 minutes a day	2-3
Friday	Strolling-Walk 10 minutes 3× a day or 30 minutes a day	2-3
Saturday	Rest	
Sunday	Rest	

Your Next Steps—If you are ready, advance yourself to the next week recommendations:

Week 2: Your goal for week #2 is to complete five days of "Strolling" accumulating a total of 30-35 minutes a day. Increase your intensity to a level 3 during your walks.

Week 3: Your goal for week #3 is to complete five to six days of "Strolling" accumulating a total of 35-40 minutes a day maintaining an intensity of a level 3-4 during your walks.

Week 4: Your goal for week #4 is to complete six to seven days of "Strolling" accumulating a total of 40 minutes a day, increasing your intensity to a level of 3-5 during your walks.

Week 5 and beyond: Continue to perform Week #4 recommendations or advance yourself to "Rolling," "Burning," or "Toning" or one of the other Walking 4 Wellness plans found in Chapters 3-6.

*Remember, to avoid plateaus, it is very important to always challenge your body by walking faster, longer or more days.

Walking 4 Your Body

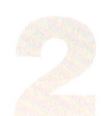

Walking 4 Your Body Workout #2: "Rolling"

Goal—Increase your walking speed and intensity:

✓ Be purposeful when "rolling;" think of being very late to a meeting and trying to catch up to someone.

✓ One of the best ways to increase the calories you burn during your walk is to increase your speed. To get you "rolling" one trick to increase your foot speed; simply increase the speed of your arms and your feet will follow.

✓ Remember to "roll" your heel to toe, walking as quickly as you can.

✓ Remember to tighten your "tush" as you walk.

✓ Before your week begins, make it a point to plan the day and time you will "roll."

✓ On a scale of 1-10, 1 = Easy light breathing, 5 = Somewhat winded and 10 = All out effort, racing someone full speed. Perform "rolling" at a 5-7 intensity level.

"Rolling" Walking For Your Body Workout—Week 1 Goal: Five days per week.

☀ DAY	🕐 WALKING WORKOUT	☰ INTENSITY
Monday	Rolling 30 minute walk	5-6
Tuesday	Strolling 30-45 minute walk	4-5
Wednesday	Rolling 30 minute walk	5-6
Thursday	Strolling 30-45 minute walk	4-5
Friday	Rolling 30 minute walk	5-6
Saturday	Rest	
Sunday	Rest	

Your Next Steps—If you are ready, advance yourself to the next week recommendations:

Week 2: Your goal for week #2 is to alternate "Rolling" three days a week with "Strolling" two to three days a week—completing five to six total days. But now, you'll want to increase your "Rolling" walk to 30-35 minutes each day and increase your intensity to a level 6.

Week 3: Your goal for week #3 is to continue to alternate "Rolling" three days a week with "Strolling" two to three days a week—completing five to six total days of walking. But, increase your "Rolling" walk to 35-40 total minutes each day and maintain your intensity at a level 6.

Week 4: Your goal for week #4 is to increase the number of days you "Roll" now performing four days a week and "Strolling" two to three days a week—completing six to seven total days of walking. Also, increase your "Rolling" walk to 40-45 total minutes each day and increase your intensity to a level 6-7.

Week 5 and beyond: Continue to perform week #4 recommendations or advance yourself to "Burning" or "Toning" or one of the other Walking 4 Wellness plans found in Chapters 3-6.

*Remember, to avoid plateaus, it is very important to always challenge your body by walking faster, longer or more days.

Walking 4 Your Body Workout #3: "Burning"

"Burning" is also known as interval training and it is one of the most effective strategies to burn fat and improve fitness levels. Studies demonstrate interval training can actually burn up to nine times more body fat when compared to slow aerobic exercise. Also, one of the many advantages of "burning" is you can accomplish more in less time. If you want to get a great workout in less time, try one of the "Burn" techniques below:

Fast Burn: Alternate between one minute of moderate-paced walking and one minute of fast-paced walking for a total of 20 or 30 minutes. For example:

FAST BURN WALK	TIME	INTENSITY
Warm-up	Minute 1:00-5:00	2-3
Moderate-paced for one minute	Minute 5:00-6:00	5-6
Fast-paced for one minute	Minute 6:00-7:00	7
Alternate between moderate-paced and fast-paced every minute	Minute 7:00-27:00	Moderate: 5, Fast: 7
Cool down	Minute 27:00-30:00	2-3

Intense Burn: If you are up to it physically and you really want to boost your fat burning ability, try an "Intense Burn" workout, alternating every 30 seconds between a fast walk and a fast jog/run. For example:

INTENSE BURN WALK	TIME	INTENSITY
Warm-up	Minute 1:00-5:00	2-3
Fast-paced for 30 seconds	Minute 5:00-6:30	6-7
Fast jog/run for 30 seconds	Minute 5:30-6:00	7-8
Alternate between fast-paced walking and fast-paced running every 30 seconds	Minute 6:00-27:00	Fast-paced walking: 6-7, Fast-paced running: 7-8
Cool down	Minute 27:00-30:00	2-3

(Continued on page 46.)

Walking 4 Your Body

Walking 4 Your Body Workout #3: "Burning" *(Continued)*
Goal—

✓ **Hill or Stair Intervals:** If you'd like to mix it up, you can also use a hill or stairs and walk, jog or run up at a fast pace and walk down slowly to recover and catch your breath, then repeat for the recommended duration.

✓ Remember, on a scale of 1-10, 1 = Easy light breathing, 5 = Somewhat winded and 10 = All out effort, racing someone full speed. Perform "Burning" at a 6-8 intensity level.

"Burning" Walking For Your Body Workout—Week 1 Goal: Six days per week.

☀ DAY	🕐 WALKING WORKOUT	☰ INTENSITY
Monday	Burning—Alternate one-minute moderate walk with one-minute fast walk for 20 min.	6-7
Tuesday	Rolling—30-45 min.	5-6
Wednesday	Burning—Alternate one-minute moderate walk with one-minute fast walk for 20 min.	6-7
Thursday	Rolling—30-45 min.	5-6
Friday	Burning—Alternate one-minute moderate walk with one-minute fast walk for 20 min.	6-7
Saturday	Strolling—30-45 min.	5
Sunday	Rest	

Your Next Steps—If you are ready, advance yourself to the next week recommendations:

Week 2: Your goal for week #2 is to continue to alternate "Toning," "Burning," and "Rolling" throughout your week, completing two of each workout for a total of six workouts for the week. This week, try to increase the number of repetitions you complete for each "Toning" exercise.

Week 3: Your goal for week #3 is to continue to alternate moderate walking with fast walking three days a week, now for a total of 25-30 minutes along with "Rolling" two days a week and "Strolling" one day, completing six total days. Perform "Rolling" walk for 40-45 minutes each day maintaining your intensity to a level 6 and "Strolling" for 60 minutes.

Week 4: Your goal for week #4 is to continue to alternate moderate walking with fast walking three days a week, now for a total of 30-35 minutes, and increase your intensity to a level 7-8 with "Rolling" two days a week and "Strolling" one day, completing six total days. Perform "Rolling" walk for 45-60 minutes each day increasing your intensity to a level 6-7 and "Strolling" for 60-90 minutes.

Week 5 and beyond: Continue to perform week #4 recommendations or advance yourself to "Toning" or one of the other Walking 4 Wellness plans found in Chapters 3-6.

*Remember, to avoid plateaus, it is very important to always challenge your body by walking faster, longer or more days.

Walking 4 Your Body Workout #4: "Toning"

You'll use the same walking technique as "Burn" walking, alternating your walking speeds between moderate and fast paced but now will add a little twist. Now you'll be adding toning exercises using your body weight or portable resistance equipment throughout your walk (see below).

TONING WORKOUT	🕐 TIME	☰ INTENSITY
1 Warm-up	Minute 1:00-5:00	2-3
2 Burn—Walk for 2 minute intervals alternating 30-second moderate speed and 30-second fast speed	Minute 5:00-7:00	6-8
3 Tone—Perform as many squats as you can in one minute	Minute 7:00-8:00	5-6
4 Burn—Walk for 2 minute intervals alternating 30-second moderate speed and 30-second fast speed	Minute 8:00-10:00	6-8
5 Tone—Perform as many push-ups as you can in one minute	Minute 10:00-11:00	5-6
6 Burn—Walk for 2 minute intervals alternating 30-second moderate speed and 30-second fast speed	Minute 11:00-13:00	6-8
7 Tone—Perform as many walking lunges as you can in one minute	Minute 13:00-14:00	5-6
8 Burn—Walk for 2 minute intervals alternating 30-second moderate speed and 30-second fast speed	Minute 14:00-16:00	6-8
9 Tone—Perform as many side leg raises as you can in one minute (alternating legs)	Minute 16:00-17:00	5-6
10 Burn—Walk for 2 minute intervals alternating 30-second moderate speed and 30-second fast speed	Minute 17:00-19:00	6-8
11 Tone—Perform bench or elbow plank for one minute	Minute 19:00-20:00	5-6
12 Cool Down	Minute 20:00-25:00	2-3

(Continued on page 48.)

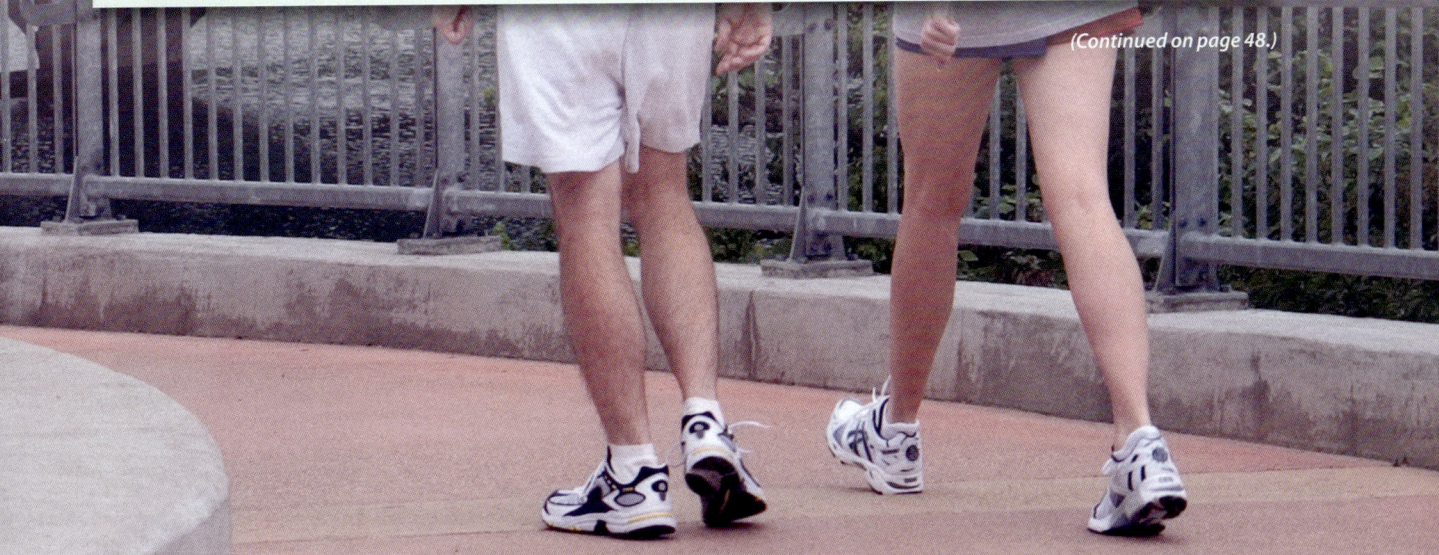

Walking 4 Your Body

4

Walking 4 Your Body Workout #4: "Toning" (Continued)

"Toning" Walking For Your Body Workout—Week 1 Goal: Six days per week.

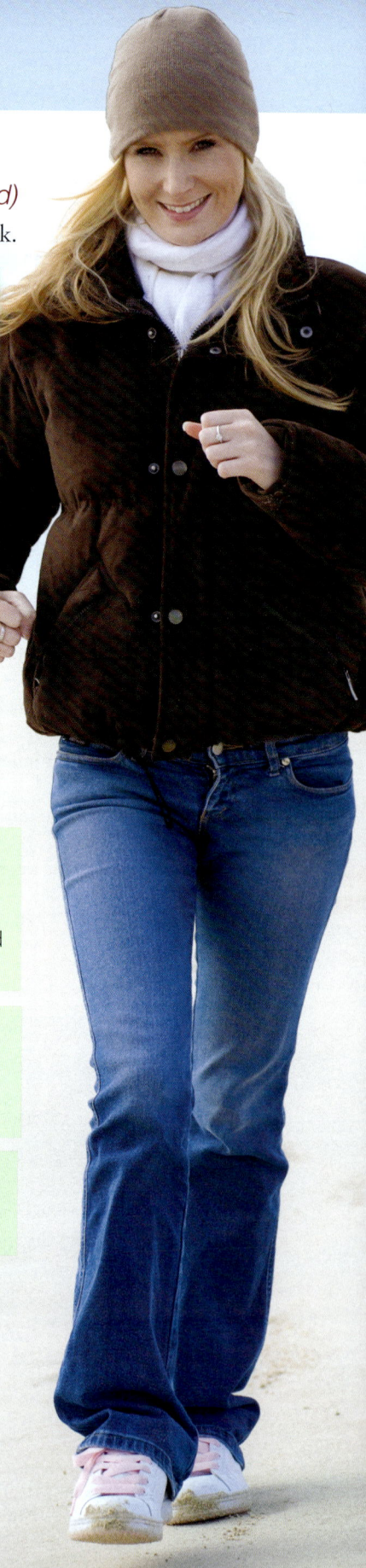

☼ DAY	🕐 WALKING WORKOUT	☰ INTENSITY
Monday	Toning—25 minutes	5-6
Tuesday	Burning—35 minutes	6-8
Wednesday	Rolling—30-45 minutes	6-7
Thursday	Toning—25 minutes	5-6
Friday	Burning—35 minutes	6-8
Saturday	Rolling—30-45 minutes	6-7
Sunday	Rest	

Your Next Steps—If you are ready, advance yourself to the next week recommendations:

Week 2: Your goal for week #2 is to continue to alternate "Toning," "Burning," and "Rolling" throughout your week, competing two of each workout for a total of six workouts for the week. This week, try to increase the number of repetitions you complete for each "Toning" exercise.

Week 3: Your goal for week #3 is to continue to alternate "Toning," "Burning," and "Rolling" throughout your week, completing two of each workout for a total of six workouts for the week. But this week, try and perform each "Toning" exercise twice. For example, perform as many push-ups as you can, take a 30 second rest and try and perform as many as you can again before moving on to the "burn" walk segment.

Week 4: Your goal for week #4 is to continue to perform two sets of each "Toning" exercise as well as adding one additional day of "Toning." Be sure to perform your "toning" workouts on non-consecutive days. (e.g. Monday, Wednesday and Friday). Feel free to drop one of your "Rolling" workouts.

Week 5 and beyond: Continue to perform week #4 recommendations or advance yourself to one of the other Walking 4 Wellness plans found in Chapters 3-6. Or go back and mix up your workouts with one of the four workouts presented.

*Remember, to avoid plateaus, it is very important to always challenge your body by walking faster, longer or more days.

Cool Toning Tools

To advance your toning program, check out the two portable tools many successful walkers have used to take their body to the next level:

1 Resistance Bands. Your portable and affordable gym! When you are on the road or at home, one of the best toning and strengthening tools is a resistance band. Not only do you get a great workout, you can simply carry your resistance bands with you and perform your toning exercises taking your fitness to another level. Resistance bands can be purchased at most sporting goods stores and come in various strengths and most are color coded, but all are very safe, convenient and affordable.

2 XCO® Walking & Running Trainer. This tool has been met with tremendous acclaim from sports and fitness enthusiasts. Runners, walkers and Nordic Walkers in particular have discovered a new sports activity for themselves. Use of the XCO-Trainer® equipment intensifies the physical benefits of normal walking and running. The integration of XCO® Walking & Running into one's normal fitness routine results in a gentle, total body workout for walkers and runners alike. With the addition of customized exercises, the scope of your workout is increased to include the development of arm and upper body strength. The result: a full body fitness routine. Unlike stationery dumbbells, specially patented granules inside help you burn more fat while you are walking or running. You can find XCO Walking and Running Trainers online at various fitness outlets and providers.

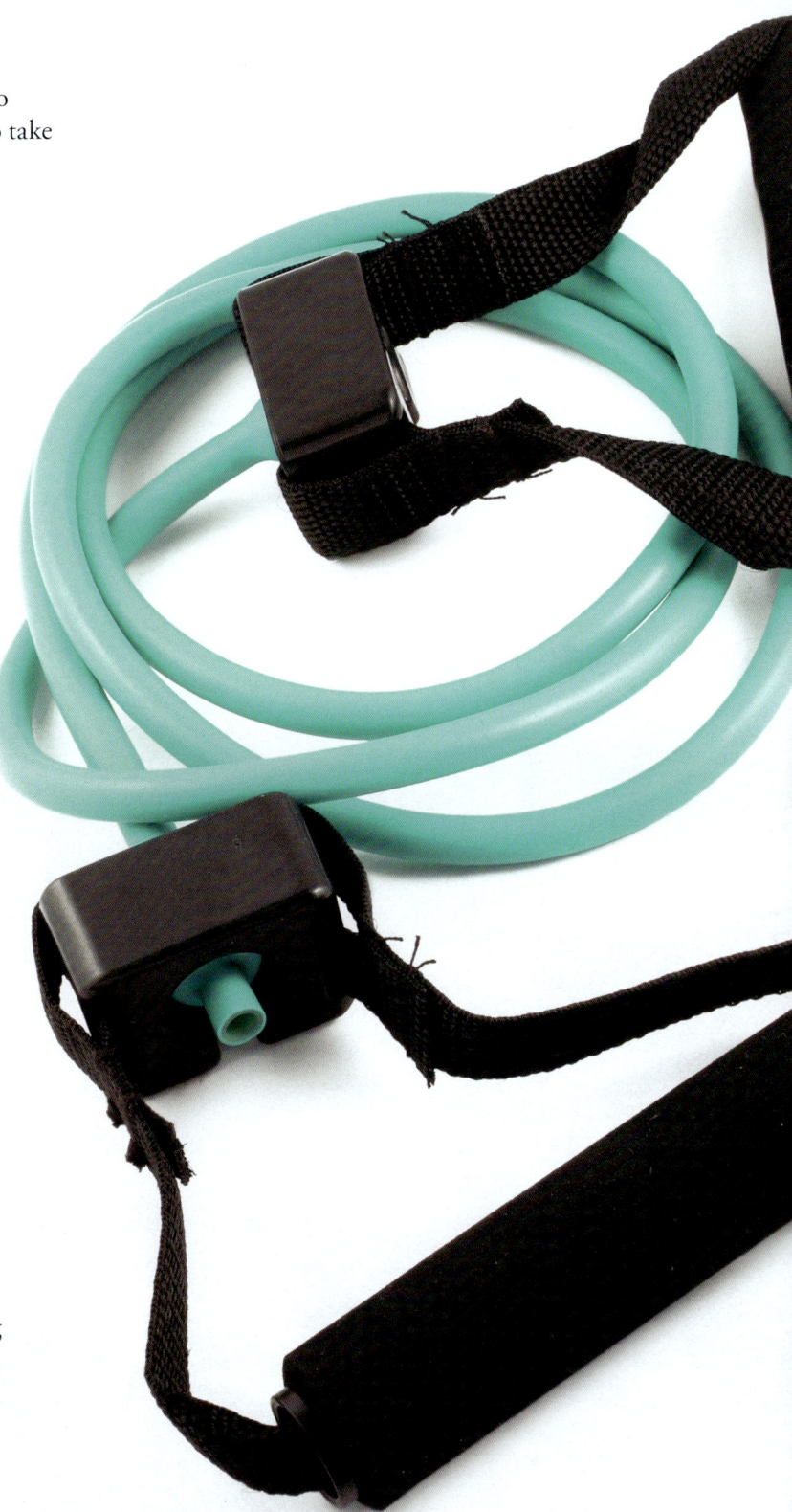

Chapter 3

Walking 4 Your Mind

Simple Steps To Combat Stress, Improve Your Mood And Put Joy In Your Step!

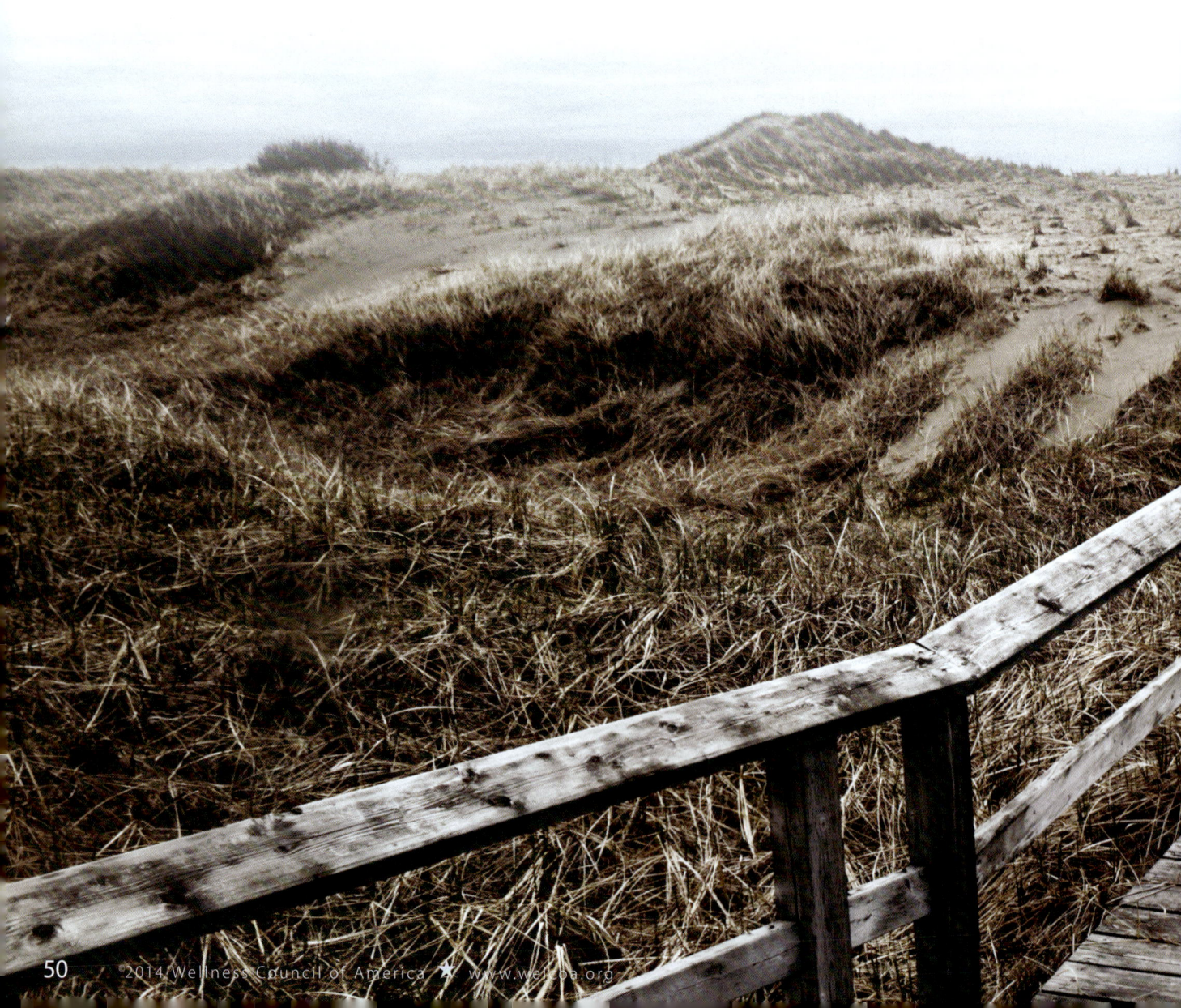

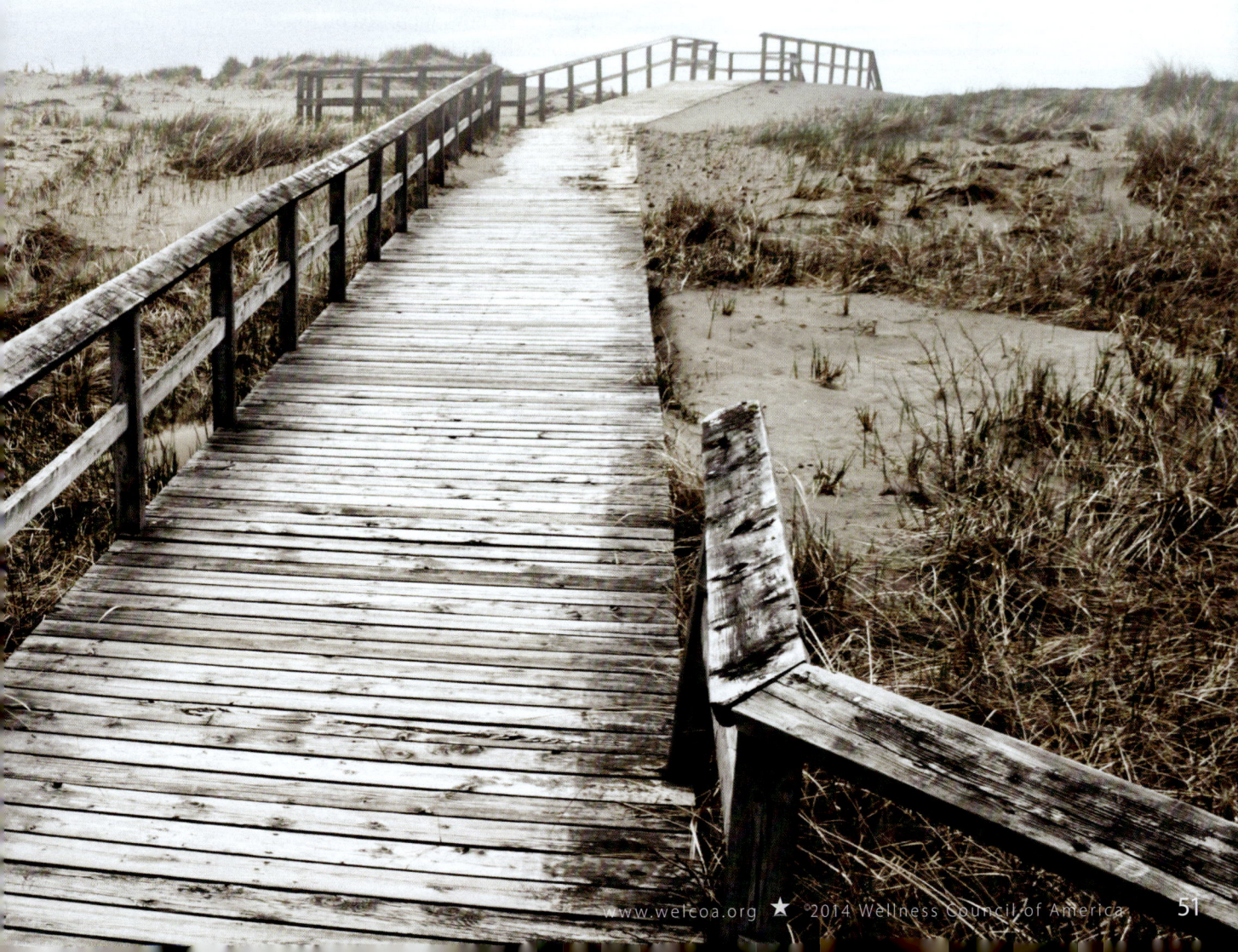

If you don't like the road you're walking,
start paving another one.

DOLLY PARTON

Walking 4 Your Mind

Spinning Plates

You probably have never heard of him before, but chances are, you've seen an example of what he did for a living. His name was Eric Brenn, and in the '50s and '60s, he was the best in the business. He was so good at what he did he made it on national television and inspired a generation of performers. It was February, 1969 when Brenn made his national debut on the famous Ed Sullivan Show. He appeared on stage in a snazzy black suit and bow tie with a stack of dinner plates in his arms along with a number of long sticks. Then with a coy smile and a wave of his hand, loud circus music began to play as he carefully set one plate on top of a wooden stick and spun it with the flick of his finger. He repeated this with two, three, four and five plates, all now, mounted on top of sticks on a dinner table, all spinning in rhythmic unison. The audience was thrilled! Brenn, the consummate showman, smiled from ear to ear, bowed to the camera and studio audience taking in their thunderous applause. But this was only the beginning. Brenn's respite was short as the plates began to wobble. Still smiling, Brenn motioned to the audience as to excuse himself and began to run back and forth spinning all the plates, busily trying to keep them from crashing to the floor. If that wasn't enough, he then began to spin additional dinner plates on top of the table where the sticks were mounted. Eight additional dinner plates now were spinning like tops along with the five others. Fourteen plates in all. The applause from the crowd was deafening, as Brenn smiled, then hurriedly yet masterfully, ran back and forth to his spinning, wobbling plates.

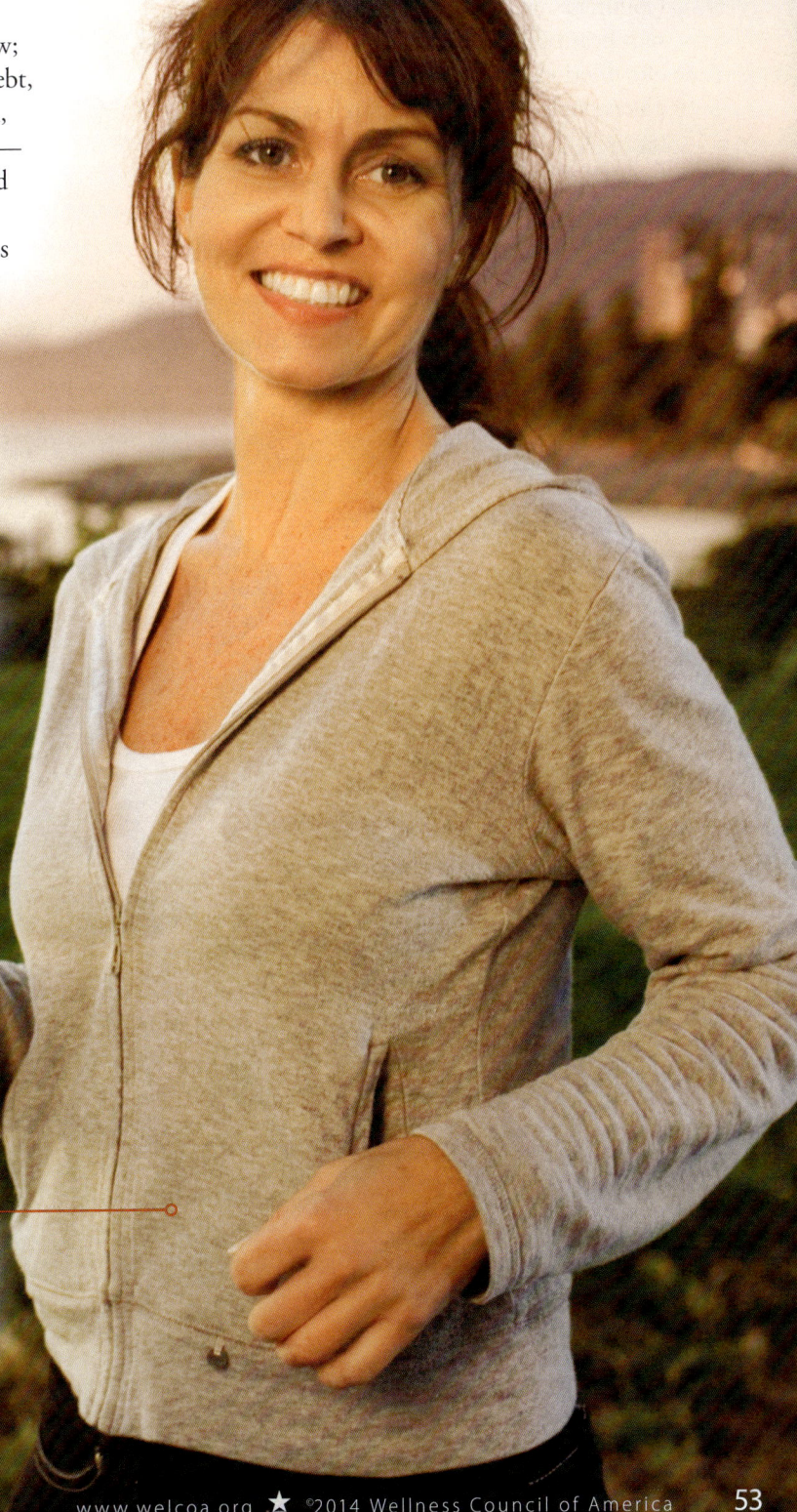

Do you ever feel like Eric Brenn? Crazily running from one responsibility to another trying to keep everything up in the air, everything going? You know; work deadlines, family obligations, finances, bills, debt, charitable work, social commitments, college tuition, aging parents, medical and dental needs, car repairs—you get the picture, right? Spinning plates, exhausted and stressed, who has time to breathe or smile or for that matter go for a walk?! If you can relate, then this chapter is for you. We will explore:

1 Why Walking 4 Your Mind

2 Stressed Out To Smiling: John's Story

3 The Impact Of Chronic Stress

4 What's Your Stress?

5 Proven Stress Management Strategies

6 Walk Well: Moving For Your Mood

7 Cool Walking Tools

In this chapter you'll learn how walking for your mind may be one of the very best things you can do to manage your stress and boost your mood and a lot more, helping you to keep on smiling as you masterfully keep all the plates spinning in your life.

Countless research studies show that walking has a significant impact on not only our bodies but also our emotional, intellectual and mental well-being.

Walking 4 Your Mind

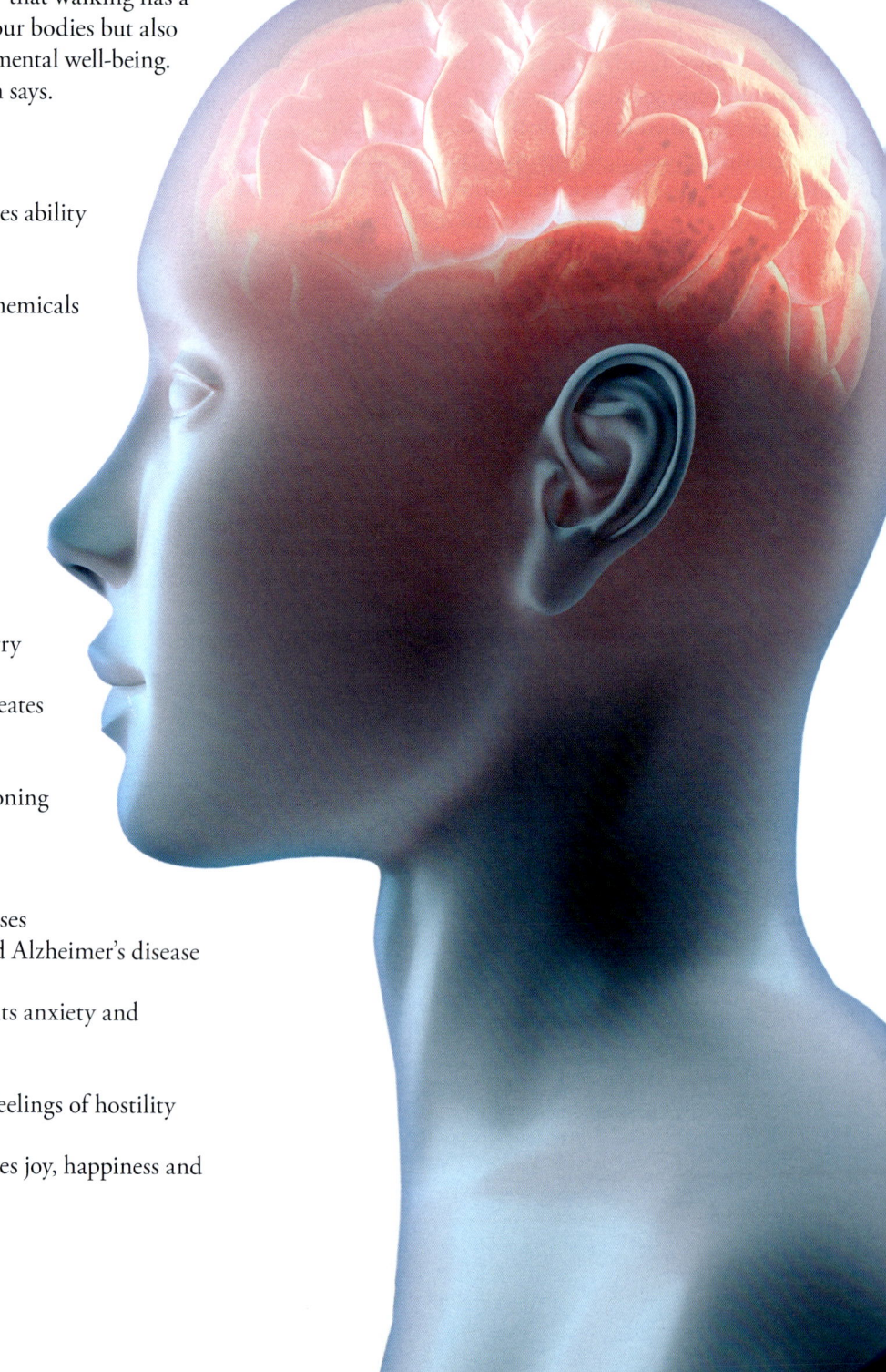

Why Walking 4 Your Mind

Countless research studies show that walking has a significant impact on not only our bodies but also our emotional, intellectual and mental well-being. Take a look at what the research says.

Regular walking:

✓ Reduces stress and improves ability to cope

✓ Releases feel-good brain chemicals like endorphins

✓ Decreases depression

✓ Alleviates symptoms of Pre-Menstrual Syndrome in women

✓ Enhances relaxation

✓ Decreases tension and worry

✓ Boosts brain power and creates new brain cells

✓ Improves cognitive functioning

✓ Enhances memory

✓ Keeps brain young, decreases symptoms of dementia and Alzheimer's disease

✓ Reduces, treats and prevents anxiety and panic attacks

✓ Helps manage anger and feelings of hostility

✓ Boosts your mood; increases joy, happiness and sense of well-being

And the list goes on and on…

Stressed Out To Smiling

John was going through the wringer. He was overworked, overweight, over-traveled, overstressed and overdue for a break. He shared with me, "Life just keeps coming so fast. I can't seem to juggle all that is thrown my way!" John had come to see me to discuss his lack of motivation to work out and his weight struggles. I asked him what had changed over the last year and he began to share what was really on his mind. "I feel like I just can't catch a break. I used to feel confident and on top of everything, including my exercise routine, but now I am floundering. I have no time to rest, no time to work out. I am jumping from one fire to another. Work is over the top! Then when I go home I try to get a workout in but there are so many needs at home. I want to be there for my wife and kids but my mind keeps racing back to all that needs to be taken care of at work. The only solace I have found is drinking a few beers when I get home and eating whatever I get my hands on. I even started taking medication for this anxiety I'm feeling." I could see the pain in John's eyes as he shared.

I encouraged him to consider ditching the idea of just "working out for the body" and consider "walking for his mind" instead. I shared the idea of walking as the best "emotional medicine" for your brain to help you just feel good. I also went on to share the many benefits to his emotional and mental well-being and gave him the tips you'll read about in this chapter. After just a few months, John, visibly lighter, happier and smiling came to tell me something that had stuck with him and I hope will stick with you. He said, "Sean, I realize I have a choice about how I look at stress. I ditched the idea of working out just for my body. I'm doing it for my sanity! Walking is the best brain medicine in the world! I wouldn't miss it for the world—it's completely changed the way I feel! My wife told me just the other day, "Honey, ever since you have been walking you are a different man. It's so nice to see your smile again!" While work is still very busy and life plates keep spinning, John is a different man. He now has a smile on his face and has found his stride. Here's hoping you find yours too.

While work is still very busy and life plates keep spinning, the idea of walking is the best "emotional medicine" for your brain to help you just feel good.

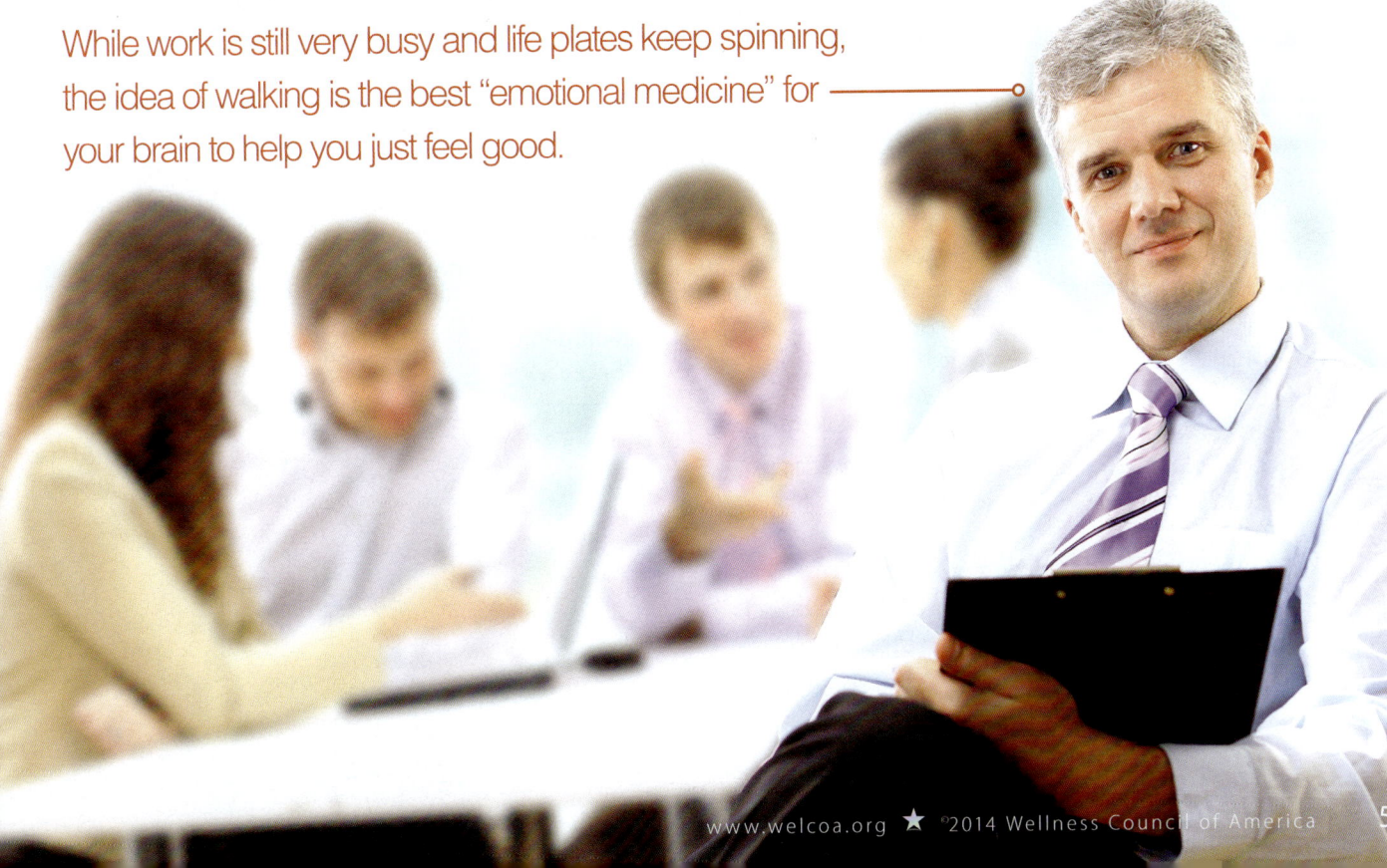

Walking 4 Your Mind

Chronic Stress

When we are constantly spinning plates, feeling worn out, anxious, frazzled or overwhelmed, contending with constant stress, the effects to our body, brain and health can be very unpleasant as well as potentially dangerous. Researchers are now beginning to crack the code in understanding how a life filled with chronic unrelenting stress leads to not only physical challenges but also emotional and life challenges as well. Author, physician and Harvard University health educator Dr. Deborah Sichel in her ground breaking book *Woman's Moods* makes this profound observation about the mind and the impact of stress: "The brain is the major organ of the body, yet it is sadly mistreated and ignored in the area of well-being and health. Without paying attention to your brain, all aspects of your life—emotional, physical and spiritual—will suffer."

Dr. Sichel's observations are directly in line with researchers at Yale, Penn State, Wake Forest, Columbia Universities and countless other physicians, scientists and health educators who have identified chronic stress being responsible for at least 80% of our health problems. Problems such as:

- ✓ Anger
- ✓ Anxiety
- ✓ Arthritis
- ✓ Cancer
- ✓ Concentration impairment
- ✓ Depression
- ✓ Decrease in muscle tissue
- ✓ Decrease in bone density
- ✓ Digestive problems
- ✓ Fatigue
- ✓ Forgetfulness
- ✓ Heart disease
- ✓ High blood pressure
- ✓ Higher risks of stroke
- ✓ Inactivity
- ✓ Feelings of burnout, fear and insecurity
- ✓ Shrinking brain and impaired cognitive function
- ✓ Increased abdominal fat
- ✓ Irritability
- ✓ Lung disease
- ✓ Metabolic Syndrome
- ✓ Over-eating
- ✓ Pre-mature aging cells
- ✓ Restlessness
- ✓ Relational discord and fighting
- ✓ Sadness
- ✓ Social isolation
- ✓ Sleep issues
- ✓ Smoking
- ✓ Suppressed thyroid function
- ✓ Under-eating
- ✓ Weight gain
- ✓ Addictive behavior (alcohol, drugs, tobacco, etc.)
- ✓ Lowered immunity, increasing incidents of illness and sickness

Here's The Good News

For most of us, stepping away from the spinning plates of life is not a realistic strategy. So how do we manage our stress and help heal and strengthen our mind? "Rewire your brain," says Laurell Mellin, clinical professor at University of San Francisco School of Medicine and New York Times best selling author. In her book, *Wired For Joy* Mellin states, "Over the last 20 years, research has shown that the source of most of our stress is in the brain itself. Given the onslaught of stress in daily life, it can easily become wired to favor stress…" Mellin has spent the last 30 years studying and making major breakthroughs in neuroscience indicating that we can use our mind, our emotions and our thinking to change our brains and our stress. Mellin adds, "The human brain has an amazing capacity to create joy not by chance but by choice."

Along with emotional and mental exercises inspired by Mellin and others, which we will look at in a moment, other researchers have identified one of the best ways to help "create joy," naturally decreasing stress and rewiring your brain is to walk or exercise regularly. According to medical doctor and professor, Dr. Marc Siegel of NYU School of Medicine: "Exercise improves blood flow to the brain, it helps the body detoxify, it puts you on a better cycle of physical behavior, and it leads to decreased stress. It also improves thinking and mental function and decreases your tendency toward addiction." And best of all, walking makes us feel good. Don't we all need a little bit more of that?

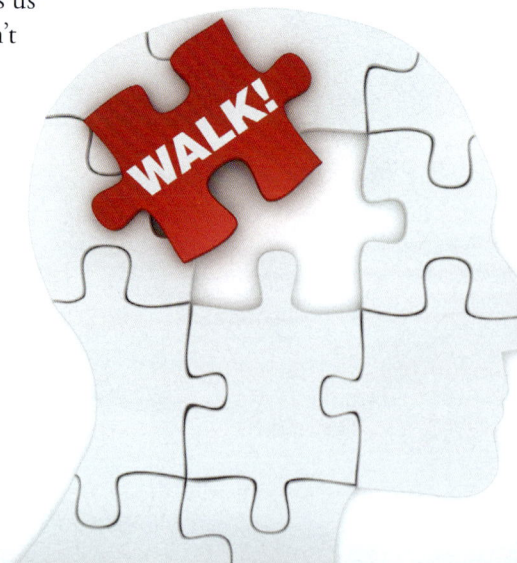

Getting Started: Ask The Right Mind Questions

Below, are a list of questions to help you determine how you are presently managing your stress by rejuvenating, renewing and strengthening your mind. You can use this tool to assess and reassess your stress coping skills as well as the potential progress you may be making with your Walking 4 Your Mind program. The questions below ask you about how frequently you practiced the following during the last week. Write down **how often** you practiced each by rating yourself (**0 = Never, 1 = Almost Never, 2 = Sometimes, 3 = Fairly Often and 4 = Very Often**).

Ask yourself, "In the last week, how often have I managed my stress by:

1. Receiving adequate rest and relaxation to feel rejuvenated _____

2. Planning ahead and managing my time well _____

3. Setting realistic goals and expectations of myself _____

4. Enjoying leisure activities, hobbies or outside interests that bring a personal sense of joy and fulfillment. _____

5. Taking responsibility for my personal commitments _____

6. Acknowledging, experiencing and constructively expressing my emotions _____

7. Speaking honestly and gracefully to myself _____

8. When challenged or in conflict, looking for ways to grow personally _____

9. Focusing on what I can control and letting go of what I can't _____

10. Thinking optimistically about my life _____

STRENGTHENING MY MIND				
Very Low	**Low**	**Average**	**High**	**Very High**
0-10	11-20	20-29	29-34	35-40

If you scored very low, low or average this week you may want to consider implementing one or more of the following tips and techniques along with your Walking 4 Your Mind program.

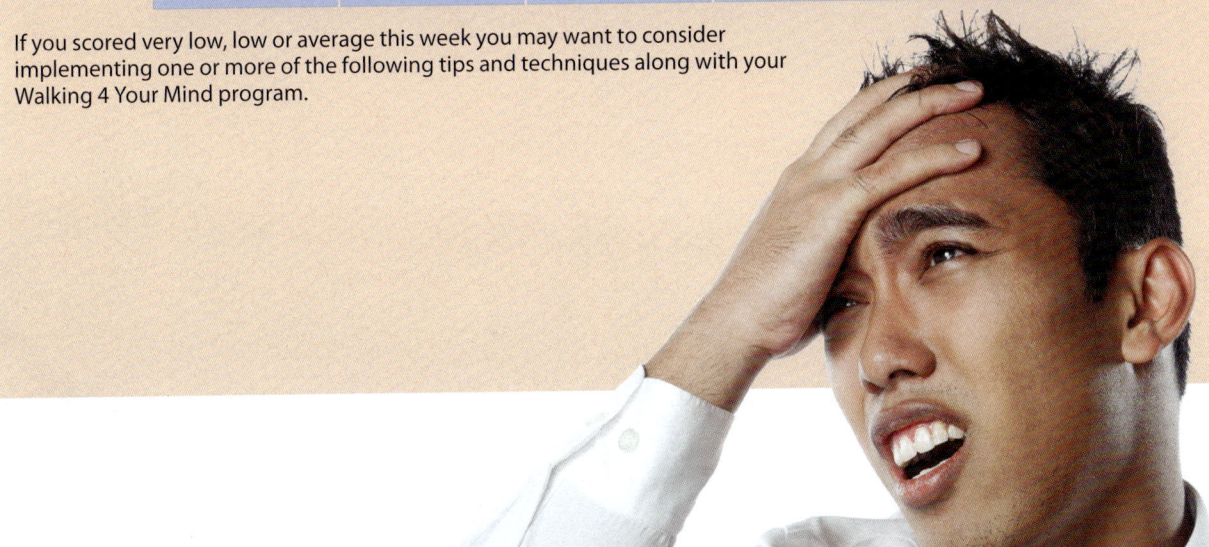

Strong Body = Strong Mind

According to research, walking not only reduces stress it can also boost your brain power—creating new brain cells and improving overall brain performance. Thomas Jefferson was right, "A strong body makes the mind strong."

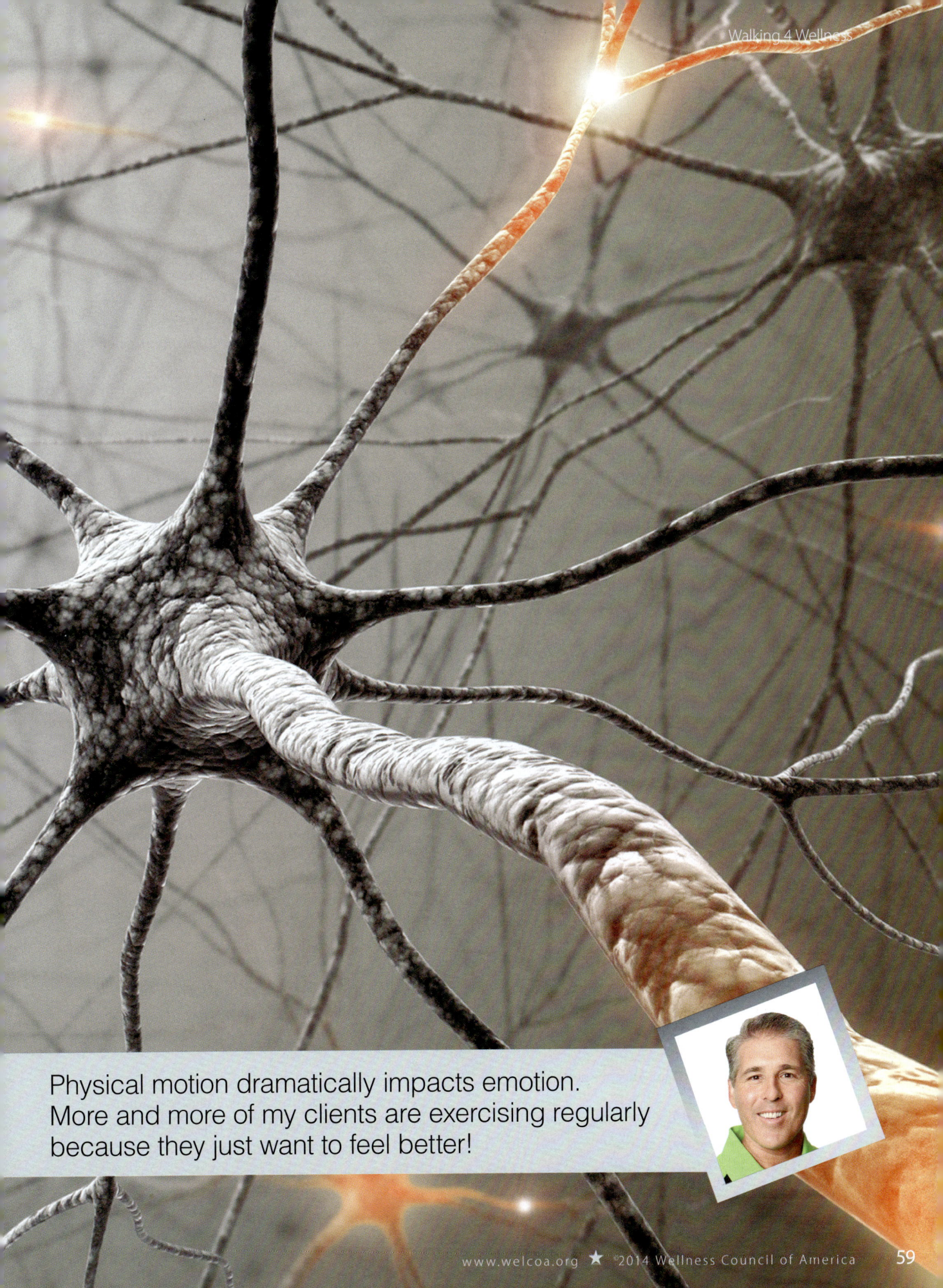

Physical motion dramatically impacts emotion.
More and more of my clients are exercising regularly
because they just want to feel better!

Walking 4 Your Mind

Walk Well: Walking 4 Stress Management And Improving Your Mood

Researchers have uncovered one of the most powerful reasons and possibly the most attainable reason to move more: to improve our mood. That's right. If you want to feel good, go for a walk! When we move we feel better. I like to say, "motion affects emotion." But did you also know you can multiply the power of motion and impact your emotions by adding just a few stress management strategies to your walking routine? According to leading researchers in the field of stress management and emotional well-being, the following four strategies will help boost your mood, mind and health!

1 ENGAGE IN DEEP BREATHING EXERCISES BEFORE OR AFTER YOUR WALK

Stress management researchers have known for years that performing deep breathing exercises is one of the best methods to tapping into the relaxation response, slowing the mind and body down and combatting chronic stress. Deep breathing exercises have been scientifically proven to increase relaxation and positively affect the brain, heart, digestion, immune system and even your genes.

A Deep Breathing: The simple act of intentionally inhaling and exhaling deeply can have a profound effect upon our relaxation response and how our brain and body respond. To help you breathe deeply place your right hand on your chest and your left hand on your abdomen and think "1, 2, 3, 4."

1. To begin breathing deeply, start by inhaling through your nose, expanding the lungs and diaphragm while mentally counting "1, 2, 3, 4."

2. Hold your breath for another count of "1, 2, 3, 4."

3. Then, slowly exhale through your mouth again and mentally count "1, 2, 3, 4."

4. Repeat this sequence and when you inhale, pay close attention to your hands. Which hand rises the most? Your right hand or your left hand? Your goal is to focus on utilizing your diaphragm when you breathe.

5. Perform this four-second breathing circuit for 1-4 minutes before or after your walk.*

6. If you'd like, you can also take your pulse before and after your deep breathing exercises to see how your deep breathing is impacting your relaxation and heart rate. (See page 65 to monitor your heart rate.)

B Resistance Breathing: By breathing in such a way that your air flow is resisted has been found in research to lower stress levels, and is called "resistance breathing." Apply the same deep breathing techniques but apply the tips below:

1. Through your nose

2. With lips pursed

3. With your tongue against the top of your mouth

4. While breathing out of a straw. By the way, this is a great conversation starter before you start your walk!

5. You can also try singing or chanting before, during or after your walk, as these are also great forms of resistance breathing

*Note: Be careful not to hold or restrict your breathing when walking as this may create light-headedness or dizziness during your walk. We recommend using deep breathing exercises before or after walks.

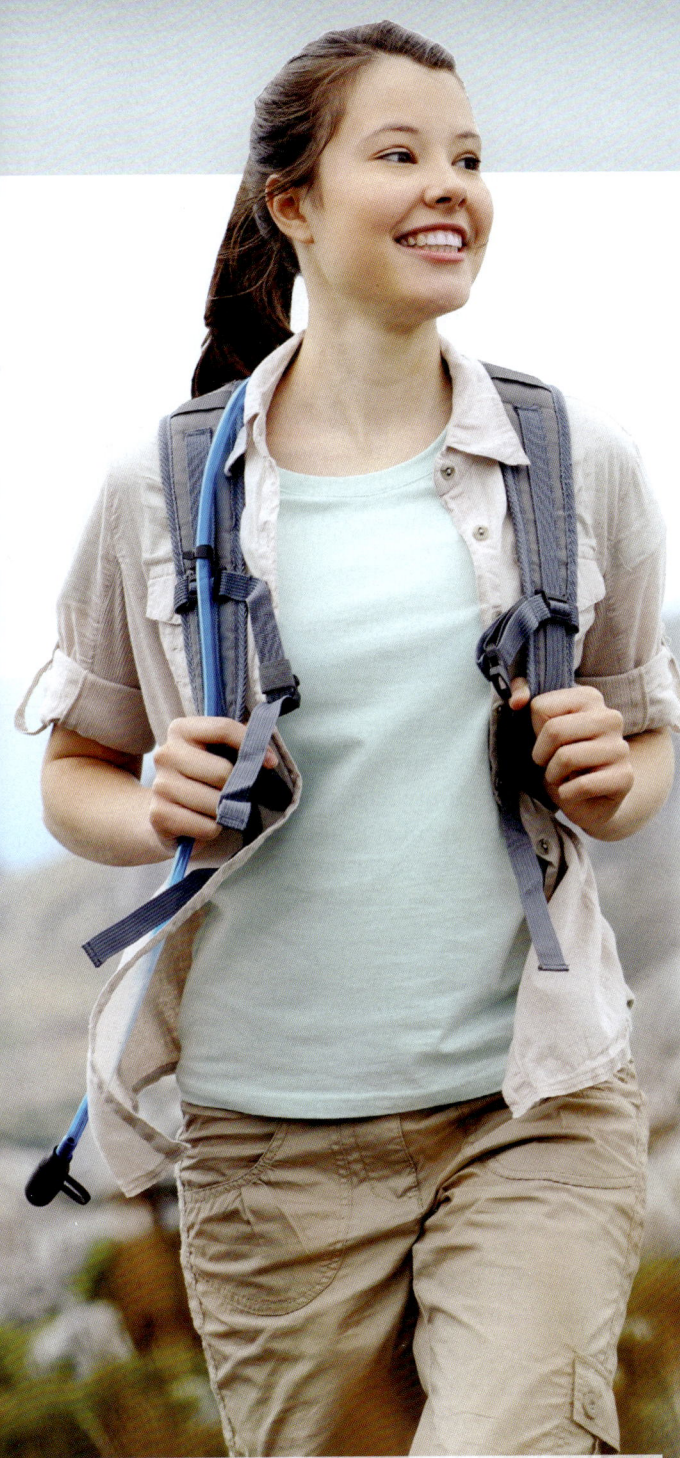

2 WALK AND TALK TO YOURSELF

Recent research in the field of psychology has discovered that using positive affirmations may not be all it is cracked up to be. Psychologists once believed that citing positive affirmations was a key to success and a cure all for managing stress and anxiety or depression. However, they are now discovering these statements may make us feel worse if we don't believe the statement, often times increasing our stress, anxiety or depression. A "third wave" of psychologists are beginning to understand how to talk to ourselves while still honoring our emotions and nurturing ourselves back to emotional well-being. Laurel Mellin along with motivational interviewing experts and acceptance and commitment therapists recommend using a series of skills when dealing with stress or challenges. You can try it for yourself. Next time you are under stress and immediately rush to tell yourself "an over the top or unbelievable affirmation" without acknowledging your present situation or emotions such as, "I never get stressed!" try the following:

A **Ask:** "How do I feel right now?

B **Feel:** Allow yourself to feel your emotions without judgment. Give yourself permission to feel and acknowledge your situation, pain or difficulty.

C **Tell:** Speak to yourself with a realistic statement of truth such as:
   ✓ "I have choices."
   ✓ "I can get help."
   ✓ "I can only do what I can do."
   ✓ "I can learn a lot from this."

Or reframe your statement in the form of a question, giving your brain a task to complete and to figure out when walking. For example, instead of saying, "I am strong and amazing!" Ask yourself, "What makes me strong and amazing?" Allow yourself the opportunity and space to feel and come up with strengths and resources you may have forgotten you possess. Ultimately, your mind will begin to search for answers to help you move in the direction you'd like to go in as well as redirecting your thoughts and managing your stress.

Self-Pep Talk!

Ultimately, your mind will begin to search for answers to help you move in the direction you'd like to go in as well as redirecting your thoughts and managing your stress.

Walking 4 Your Mind

3 **PRACTICE "LAUGH WALKING"**

Researchers agree, laughter has an incredible impact upon our body and mind and is one of the best medicines. So why not try walking and laughter together and get double the benefits? Based upon findings of Dr. Madan Kataria, and his research on the effects of laughter combined with exercise, he discovered our brain does not know the difference between a "real laugh" and a "fake laugh" and anyone can learn to laugh with just a few simple techniques. For example:

1 **Accept you don't need a reason to laugh. Just laugh—anytime, anywhere!**

2 **Before, during or after your walk:**

   a Place your hands on your stomach, while focusing on your stomach and make the sound "Ho-Ho-Ho!"

   b Next, place your hands on your chest, while focusing on your chest and make the sound "Ha-Ha-Ha!"

   c Move your hands from stomach to chest shouting, "Ho-Ho-Ha-Ha-Ho-Ho, Ha, Ha!"

   d Next, focus your attention and lay your hands on your head and make the sound, "He-He-He-He!"

   e Go back and forth between your chest, stomach and head with "Ho-Ho-Ha-Ha-Ha-He-He!"

   f Lastly, concentrate on your feet, moving them up and down as if trampling grapes and make the sounds "Hu-Hu-Hu-Hu!"

3 **It is always best to do "laugh walking" with others,** but if alone, you may want to find an area where you won't be distracted or misunderstood!

4 **Walk and talk with others:** One of the best things you can do for your mind, emotional well-being and stress management is to get a buddy to walk and talk with you. Below are a few ideas to help you walk and talk:

   a **Buddy up.** Walk with your spouse, family member or colleague at work.

   b **Join or start a walking group.** Check out all the resources at your work or in your community related to walking clubs. Usually companies, fitness facilities or gyms in your area will offer free walking clubs. If not, think about starting your own.

   c **Get a dog.** Scientists from the University of Western Australia found that people walk 48 minutes more per week after they get a dog. Dogs are a natural fitness trainer—reminding you daily to take care of yourself, encouraging you to move with every step and wag of their tail. They are also great listeners.

Walk Well: Moving For Your Mood

Now that you've learned some proven stress management strategies to help with "Walking 4 Your Mind," you are now ready to put it into practice. Below you will find a Mood Boosting routine that combines "Strolling and Rolling" along with the mentioned stress management techniques. If you'd prefer, you can also use one of the four walking styles in the previous "Body" chapter in conjunction with the mind strategies presented in this chapter. If you'd like a refresher on what type of walking is best for you go to pages 24 to 28. Be sure and select the type of walking routine you feel most confident you can accomplish and are physically ready to perform.

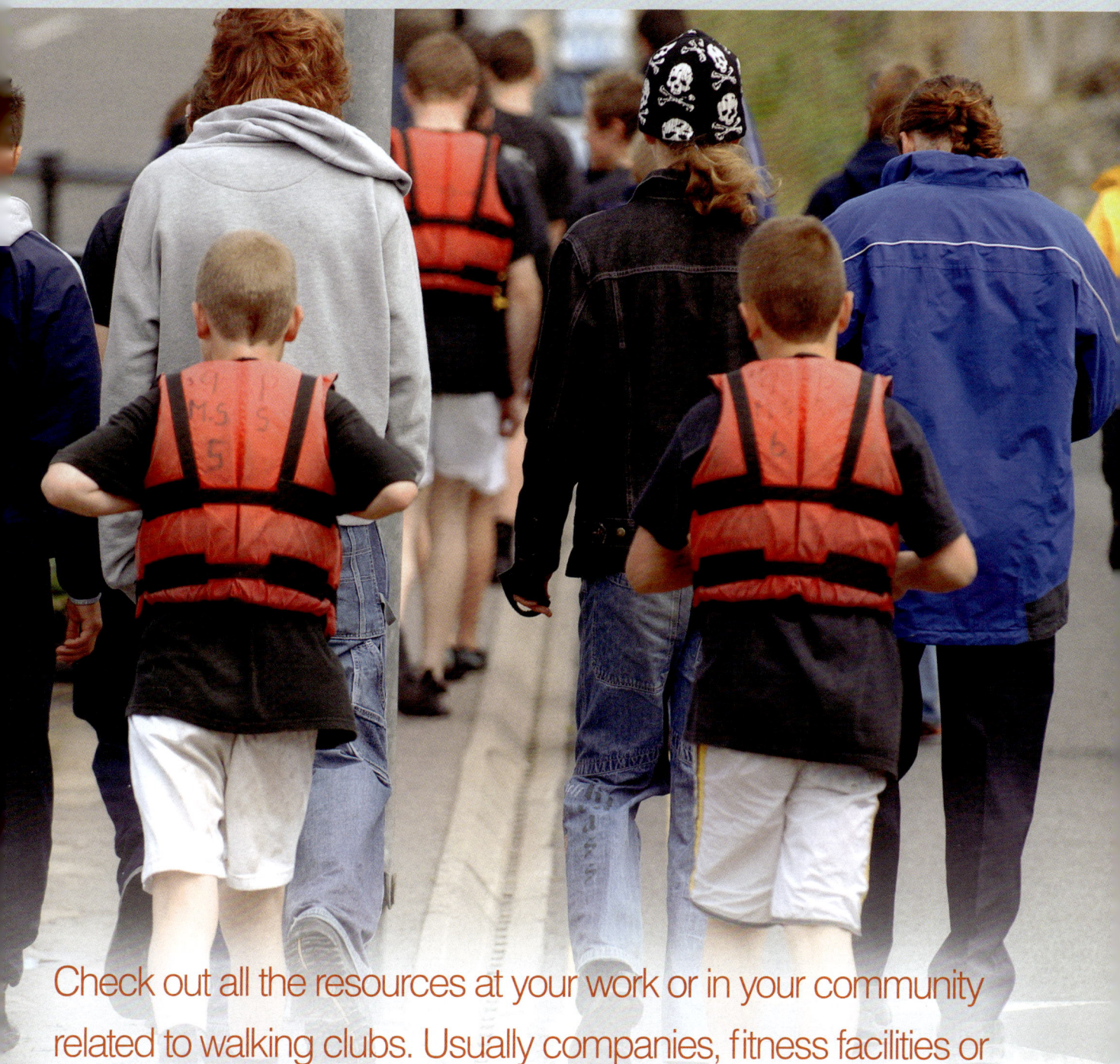

Check out all the resources at your work or in your community related to walking clubs. Usually companies, fitness facilities or gyms in your area will offer free walking clubs. If not, think about starting your own.

Walking 4 Your Mind

Walking 4 Your Mind: "Mood Booster Routine"

Goal—Enhance your mood, increase your energy and decrease your stress with this weekly walking routine.

✓ Take a 10-minute stroll at home or work just to unwind.

✓ Perform deep breathing exercises before or after your walk.

✓ Before, during or after your walk practice "Laugh Walking"—it's a hoot!

✓ Talk to yourself. Allow yourself to feel and repeat truthful, believable affirmations during your walk such as:

> ▶ "I have a choice."
> ▶ "I can only do what I can do."
> ▶ "I can get help if I need it."

> ▶ "Focus on what you can change—let go of what you can't."
> ▶ "Just take one step at a time."

✓ Enjoy some light stretching and deep breathing after your walk.

✓ When possible, walk with a buddy.

✓ On a scale of 1-10, 1 = Easy, light breathing, 5 = Somewhat winded and 10 = Racing someone full speed, almost breathless, perform "Strolling" and "Rolling" at a 2-5 intensity level.

Walking 4 Your Mind: Mood Booster Routine—Week 1 Goal: Five days per week. Focus on using breathing techniques this week, especially before or after your walks.

☀ DAY	🕐 WALKING WORKOUT	☰ INTENSITY
Monday	Strolling—Walk 10 minutes/day	2-3
Tuesday	Rolling—Walk 10 minutes/day	2-3
Wednesday	Strolling—Walk 10 minutes/day	2-3
Thursday	Strolling—Walk 10 minutes/day	2-3
Friday	Rolling—Walk 10 minutes/day	2-3
Saturday	Rest	
Sunday	Rest	

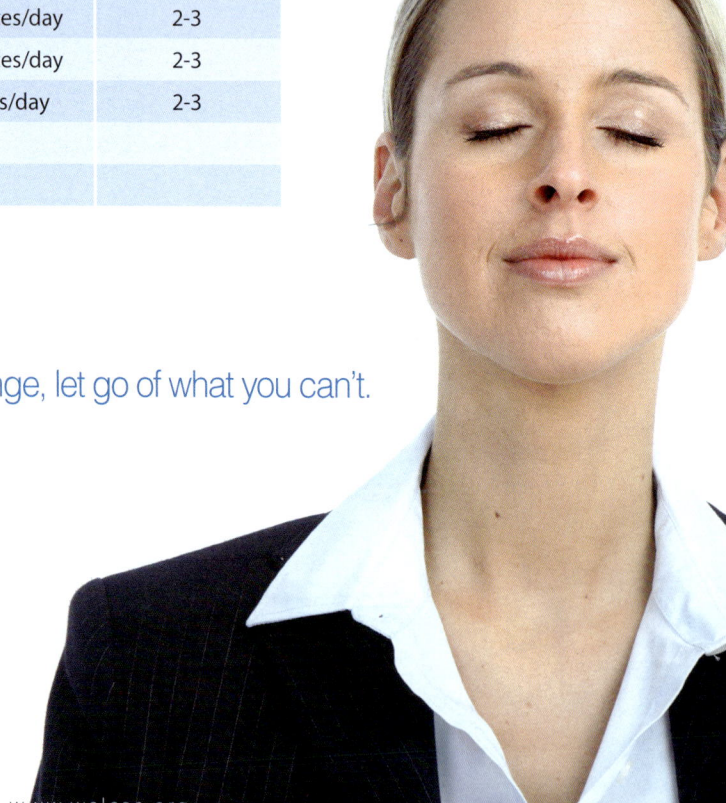

I have a choice.

Focus on what you can change, let go of what you can't.

I can only do what I can do.

Just take one step at a time.

I can get help if I need it.

Your Next Steps—If you are ready, advance yourself to the next week recommendations:

Week 2: Your goal for week #2 is to complete five days of "Mood Booster" walking, but now accumulating a total of 20 minutes a day. If you'd like you can increase your intensity to a level 3 during your walks. This week, focus on "Walking and Talking" to yourself—remembering to "Ask, Feel and Tell" yourself the truth.

Week 3: Your goal for week #3 is to complete five to six days of "Mood Booster" walking accumulating a total of 30 minutes a day maintaining your intensity of a level 3 during your walks. This week, focus on giving "Laugh Walking" a try.

Week 4: Your goal for week #4 is to complete six to seven days of "Mood Booster" walking accumulating a total of at least 30 minutes a day, increasing your intensity to a level of 3-5 during your walks. This week, focus on asking a buddy to walk and talk with you.

Week 5 and beyond: Continue to perform Week #4 recommendations and utilize the various mind and stress techniques. Or choose one of the other Walking 4 Wellness plans found in Chapters 2 and 4-6.

*Remember, to avoid plateaus, it is very important to always challenge your body by walking faster, longer or more days.

Cool Tools

To help you manage your stress and boost your mood further check out a portable tool many successful walkers have used to take their mind routines to the next level:

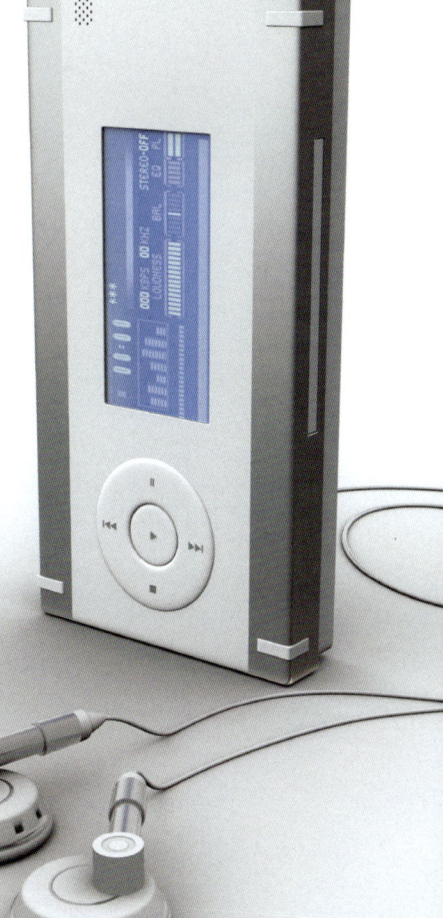

1   **MP3, iPod, Smart Phone & Headphones.** A good playlist may be just what you need to increase your joy and get you going on your Mood Booster Walk or any type of walk for that matter. Match your playlist to your mood or walking goals. Go to iTunes and download your favorite songs to fit your mood and style.

2   **Heart Rate Monitors.** Many walkers wonder "how fast should I walk?" or "how do I get the most out of my walking routine?" Both questions can best be answered by monitoring your intensity. By far the most effective way to monitor your intensity, without undue stress, is by using a cool tool called a "heart rate monitor." A heart rate monitor provides you with a reliable and convenient way to track your heart's activity.

The simplest heart rate units measure the activity of your heart. The more advanced models serve as a "virtual coach" instructing you to increase or decrease your pace. Some advanced models will also display distance covered, calories expended and have other bells and whistles such as, GPS capabilities, feedback after your workout or even can create a personal walking or jogging workouts for you based upon your personal goals and previous workouts. Heart rate monitors vary in price and function. There are many viable options when looking for a reliable heart rate monitor. I recommend my clients to use Polar® heart rate monitors. If you are interested, you can learn more about these monitors by going to your local sporting goods store or going to **polar.com**.

Chapter 4

Walking 4 Your Career & Finances

Simple Steps To Boost Your Earning Potential And Raise Your Human Capital!

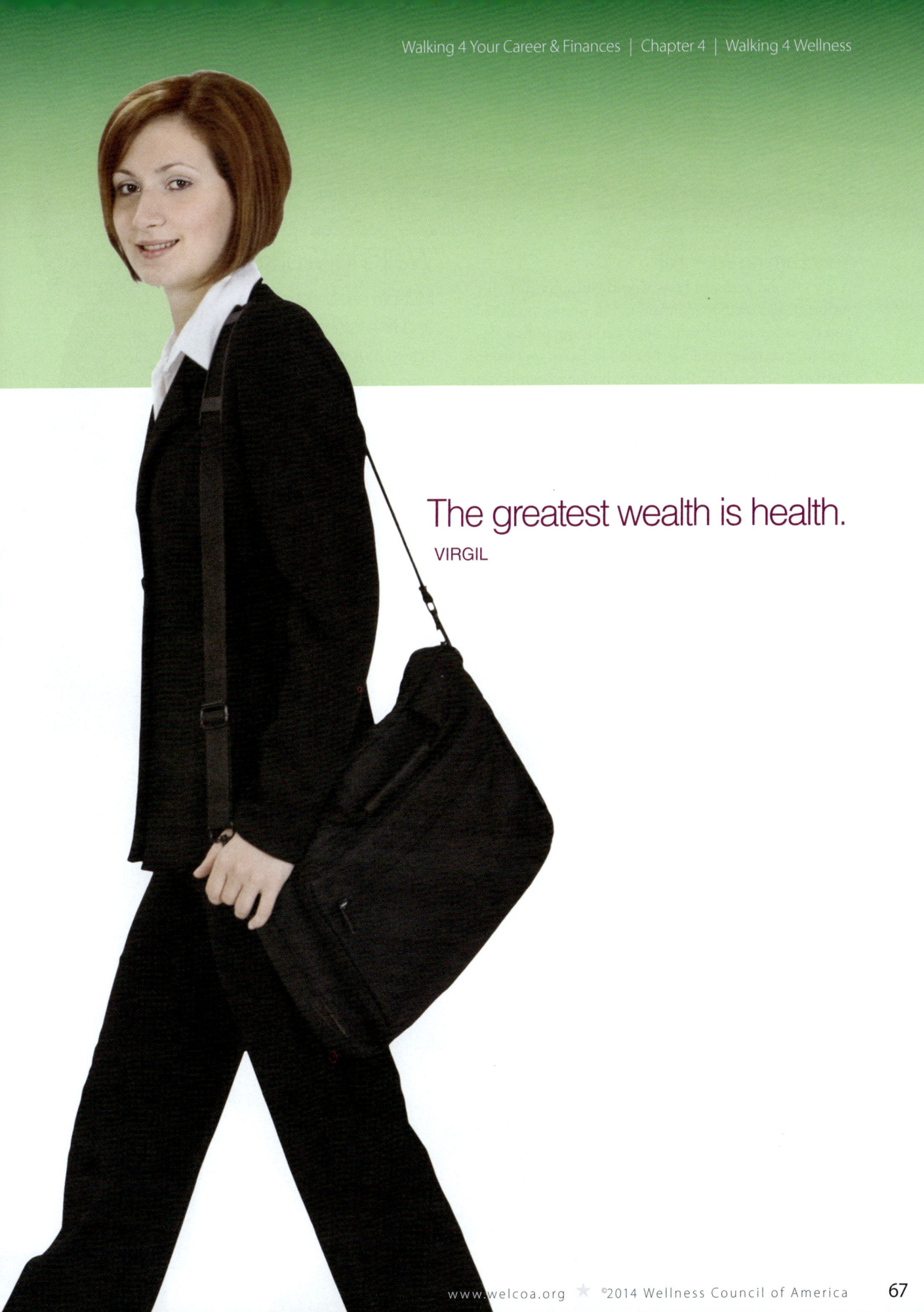

The greatest wealth is health.
VIRGIL

Walking 4 Your Career & Finan

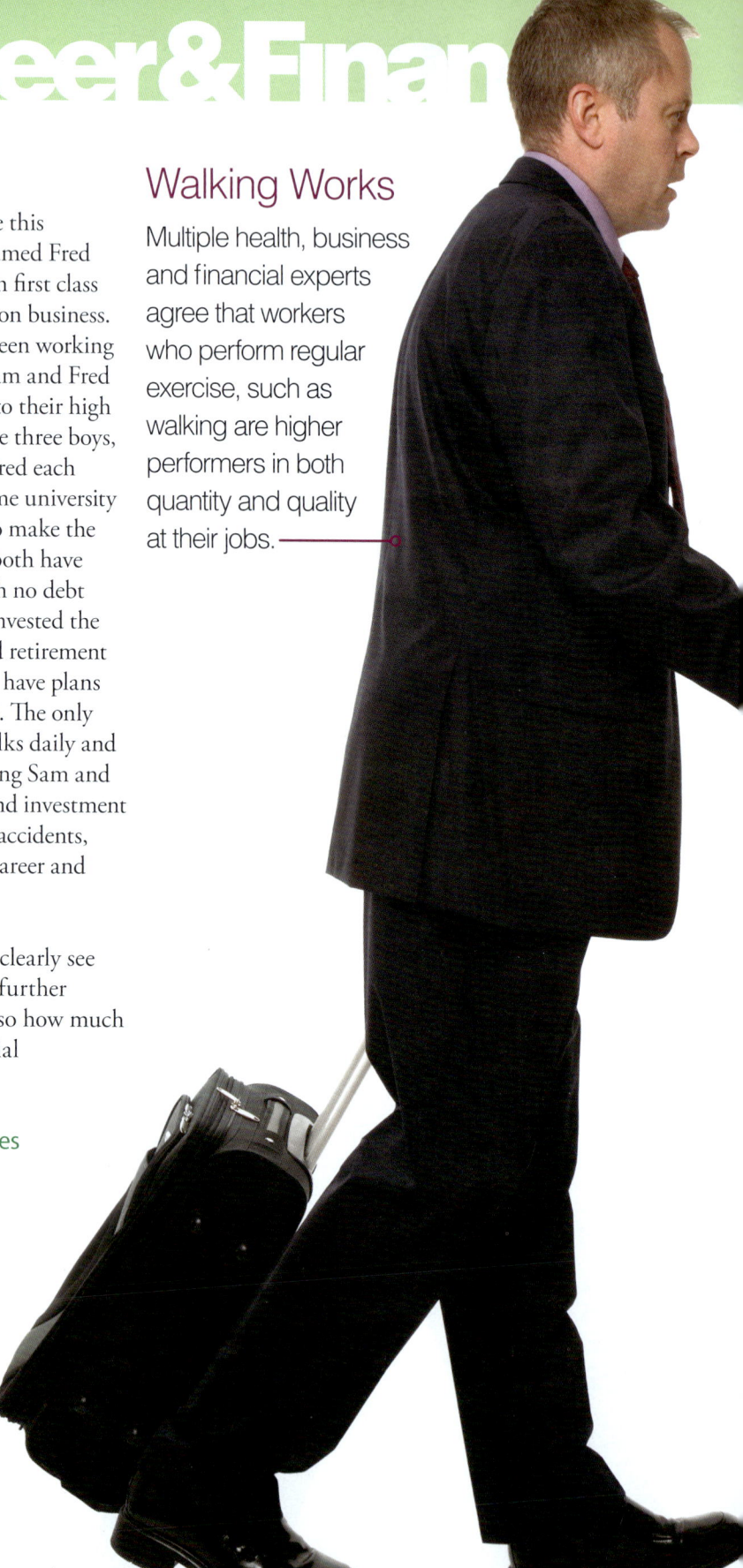

Your Earning Potential

Are you good at math? How would you solve this problem? Picture two identical twins, one named Fred and the other named Sam. Both are sitting in first class next to each other on a 747 headed to Japan on business. Both are successful businessmen who have been working in the same company for the last 15 years. Sam and Fred are 40 years old, have been happily married to their high school sweethearts for 20 years and each have three boys, identical triplets, all 10 years old. Sam and Fred each have college degrees and MBA's from the same university and both are avid readers. Sam and Fred also make the same salary, having similar jobs. They even both have the same amount of money in the bank, with no debt to their names. Believe it or not, both have invested the same amount of money into their 401k's and retirement accounts every year. Sam and Fred also each have plans to retire from their company at the age of 65. The only difference between Sam and Fred is Sam walks daily and Fred does not. Here's your question: Assuming Sam and Fred each continue their current spending and investment habits and way of living with no foreseeable accidents, who in your opinion will have the stronger career and financial future?

Not sure? By the end of this chapter, you'll clearly see the answer to this question and how much further along Sam would be at the age of 65 and also how much walking can impact your career and financial potential. In this chapter we will explore:

1 Why Walking 4 Your Career & Finances

2 Panic To Promotion: Holly's Story

3 What's Your Greatest Asset

4 Proven Human Capital Strategies

5 Walk Well: Moving For Your Career & Financial Health

6 Cool Walking Tools

Walking Works

Multiple health, business and financial experts agree that workers who perform regular exercise, such as walking are higher performers in both quantity and quality at their jobs.

Why Walking 4 Your Career & Finances

According to business analysts, productivity specialists and numerous studies, individuals who exercise are way ahead of the pack when it comes to competition. Multiple health, business and financial experts agree that workers who perform regular exercise, such as walking are higher performers in both quantity and quality at their jobs. Take a look at what the science says.

Regular walking:

✓ Improves thinking

✓ Enhances your learning, time management and judgment

✓ Boosts your creativity

✓ Increases stamina, energy and endurance

✓ Elevates self esteem, self image and confidence

✓ Increases your productivity

✓ Boosts morale

✓ Increases initiative, leadership

✓ Raises assertiveness and enthusiasm for life

✓ Reduces absenteeism and presenteeism

✓ Raises career advancement opportunities and earning potential

✓ Boosts your human capital—your health, attitude, motivation, skills, education—everything you bring to the table to make you uniquely financially valuable.

Walk 4 Your Career & Finances

You may be asking, OK I get it, walking is one of the best things I can do for my career and financial future, but aren't there other forms of exercise to also help boost my earning potential? It is true, other aerobic exercises can also help you build your human capital, but here are just a few more reasons why we think walking may just be the best exercise to help your bottom line:

1 **It's inexpensive.** One of the most common reasons cited by individuals who do not exercise regularly is the cost of exercise equipment. Well, I've got two words for you when it comes to walking: "It's Free!" Walking doesn't cost anything—just the cost of a good pair of shoes. That's good news for the budget!

2 **It's safe.** Nearly everyone from young to old to pregnant can experience the many health and fitness benefits of walking without undue strain or risk of injury—unlike many "fad" fitness systems. Talk about saving on those doctor and physical therapy bills!

3 **It's easy to do.** You don't need any special lessons, equipment or training to walk briskly and reap the many benefits to your mind, body and spirit. Again, savings galore!

4 **It's convenient.** Walking is something you can do anytime, almost anywhere. No need for special gear, gym memberships or fancy equipment, all you need is a safe area to hoof it and you are on your way. Another opportunity to save some money.

5 **It helps you market.** A healthy, happy smiling worker, salesman or leader is a great example of your company whether you work for one or own your own. Bottom line: You are your greatest sales and marketing tool. Walking will help you look physically younger and feel emotionally better, which helps you attract others to your work, product, service or cause.

Walking 4 Your Career & Finances

Panic To Promotion: Holly's Story

Holly was scared to answer the phone. Each ring twisted her stomach in knots! Would she finally get the promotion she had longed for? Taking a deep breath, Holly answered the phone. The words she dreaded to hear were spoken, "Holly, I'm sorry. We have decided to go with someone else. But we really appreciate you coming in for the interview." Holly was devastated. With mounting debt and college tuition soon approaching for her high school senior daughter, Holly wasn't sure where to go from here.

After a few weeks, she decided to seek out the help of a business coach recommended by a close friend. The day arrived for Holly's first meeting with her coach, Beth. After some pleasantries, Beth began to ask Holly a series of poignant questions: "Holly, how would you assess your

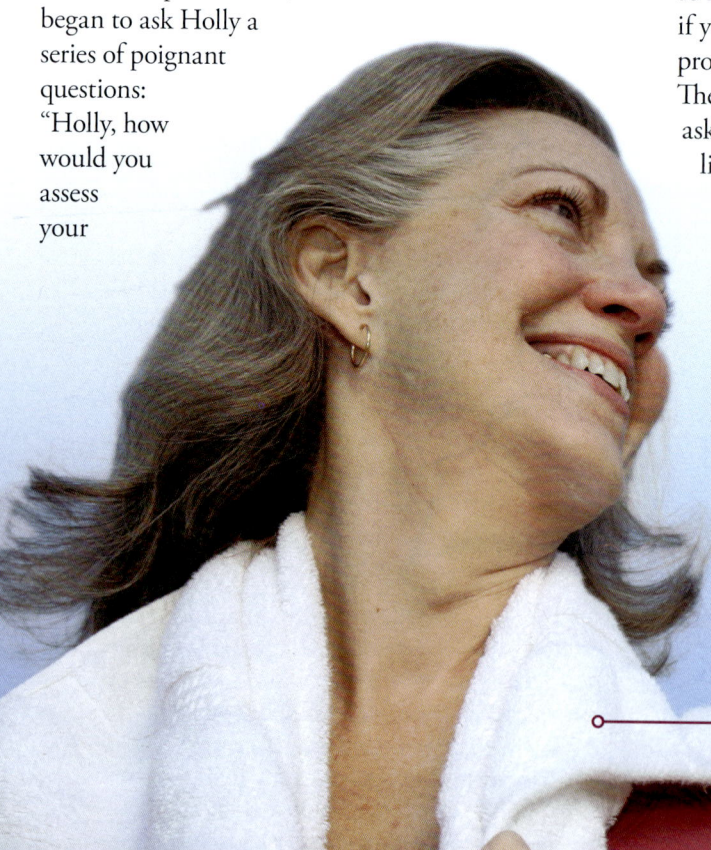

human capital?" Holly, confused, asked, "What is human capital?" Beth apologetically replied, "Oh, I'm sorry. Let me explain. Human capital is any investment you make in yourself that increases your economic value for yourself, your employer or the community. For example, investing in your education or regular exercise are two good examples of investments you can make to boost your human capital."

"Exercise? How does exercise increase my human capital?" asked Holly. Beth went on to explain all the many benefits exercise adds to your earning potential. "If there is one thing I have seen make the greatest difference over all the years I've been coaching on enhancing your productivity, morale, energy, attitude and self esteem and so much more, it's exercise. Beyond going back to school, if you want to boost your chances of getting hired, promoted or a raise, I strongly suggest you get moving!" The meeting continued for over an hour, with Holly asking questions and taking copious notes. Holly set a list of specific goals, and number one on her list was: "Start a walking program tomorrow!"

Over the next 12 weeks Holly faithfully walked at work, home and even when on vacation. Not only was she coming into work happier, more energetic, motivated, confident and with an extra bounce in her step, she also got the attention of one of the top executives when she solved a complex client issue saving the company thousands of dollars. But, here's the kicker—three weeks later, Holly was promoted to a new management position with a hefty pay raise! All of this made her daughter's high school graduation ceremony and celebration very, very special indeed!

The greatest asset you bring to a rich, secure and satisfying life is a healthy and fit YOU!

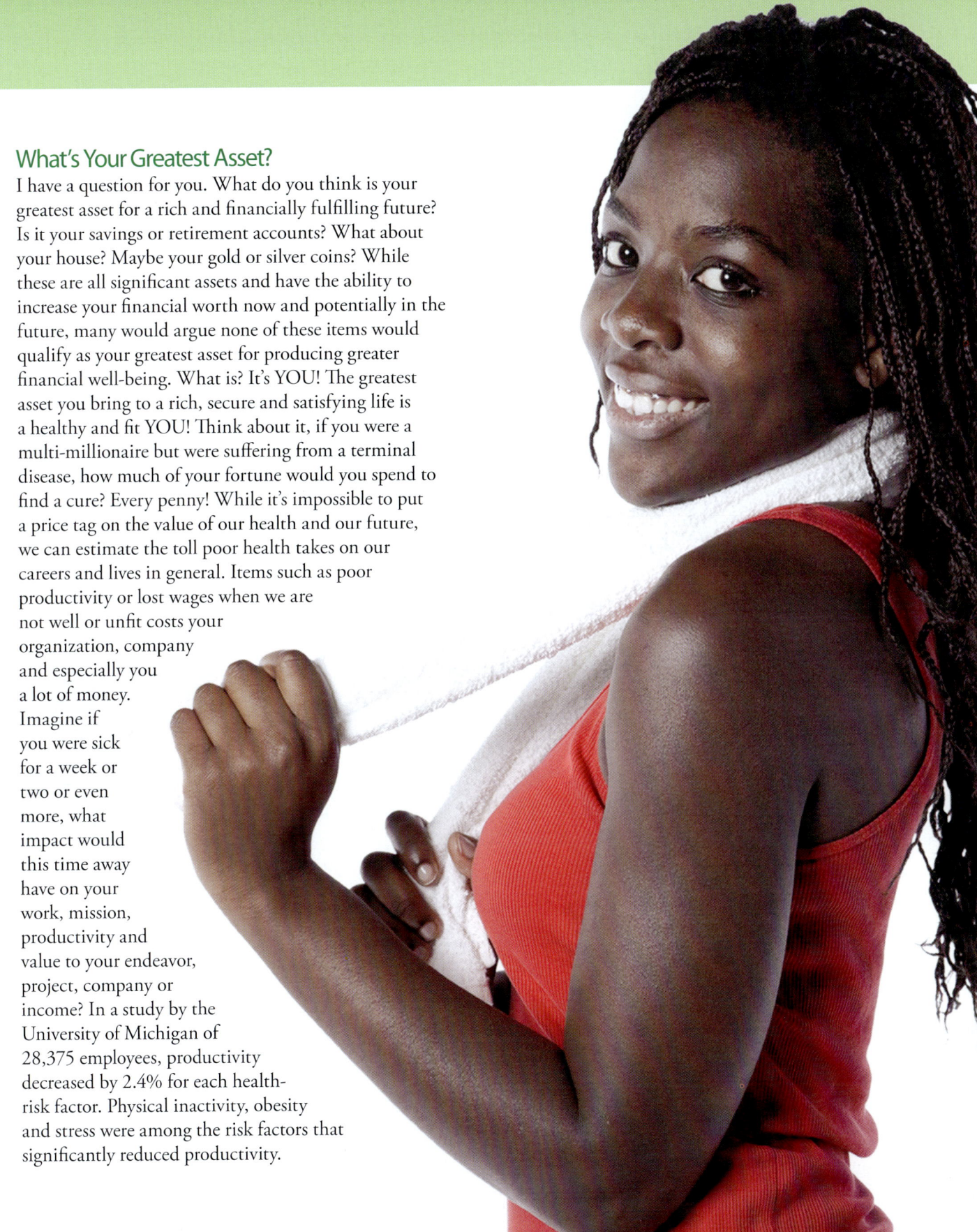

What's Your Greatest Asset?

I have a question for you. What do you think is your greatest asset for a rich and financially fulfilling future? Is it your savings or retirement accounts? What about your house? Maybe your gold or silver coins? While these are all significant assets and have the ability to increase your financial worth now and potentially in the future, many would argue none of these items would qualify as your greatest asset for producing greater financial well-being. What is? It's YOU! The greatest asset you bring to a rich, secure and satisfying life is a healthy and fit YOU! Think about it, if you were a multi-millionaire but were suffering from a terminal disease, how much of your fortune would you spend to find a cure? Every penny! While it's impossible to put a price tag on the value of our health and our future, we can estimate the toll poor health takes on our careers and lives in general. Items such as poor productivity or lost wages when we are not well or unfit costs your organization, company and especially you a lot of money. Imagine if you were sick for a week or two or even more, what impact would this time away have on your work, mission, productivity and value to your endeavor, project, company or income? In a study by the University of Michigan of 28,375 employees, productivity decreased by 2.4% for each health-risk factor. Physical inactivity, obesity and stress were among the risk factors that significantly reduced productivity.

Take Fitness Baby Steps

One of the best ways to "ease" back into a regular fitness program is to "start small." Set small realistic goals allowing you the opportunity to "fit" exercise into your daily schedule—as well as increasing your confidence as you accomplish small measurable goals.

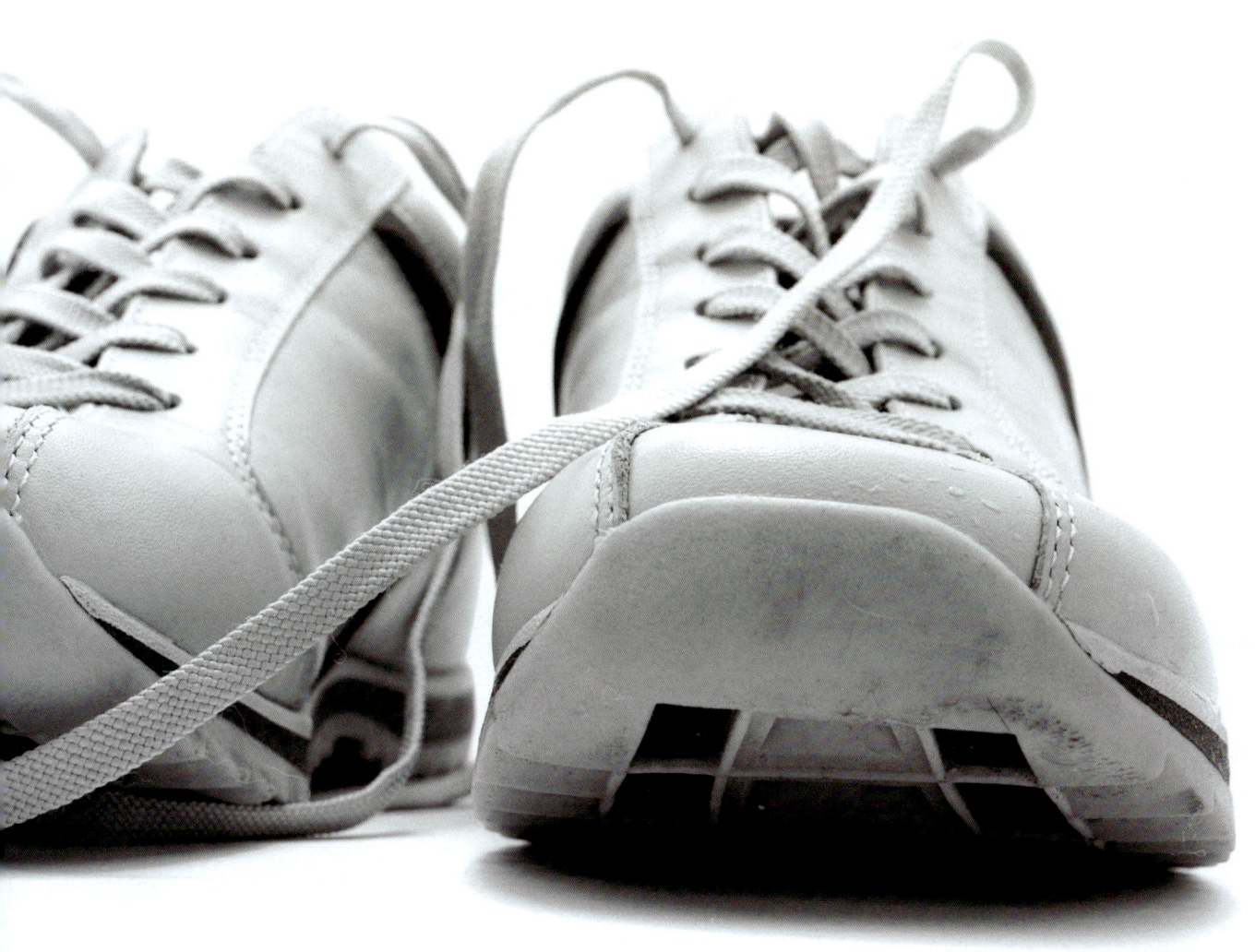

Setting small achievable goals is the key to daily success!

Walking 4
Your Career & Finances

Investing In YOU

Famed investor and billionaire, Warren Buffett once said, "The best investment you can make is always in yourself." What investments yield the greatest returns? Multiple studies show that making small investments in activities, such as regular walking can have a profound impact on your career and bottom line. Every healthy step you take is like dropping silver dollars in your "human capital" piggy bank, daily adding up for a bright and successful financial future! For example, according to the *Journal of Occupational and Environmental Medicine* employees who work out and maintain a healthy body weight have lower health care costs, fewer absences and increased productivity than inactive employees who are overweight or obese. Can you hear that little piggy bank singing? "Cha-Ching-Cha-Ching!"

Listen to what the past president of the American Medical Association, Ronald Davis, MD, had to say about the importance of being active: "Indeed, exercise is not an option, but a necessary, active, direct way that people can maintain good health, avoid illness, improve the quality of their lives, reduce their health care costs and extend their life expectancy." You know what I want to say, right? "Cha-Ching!"

> Indeed, exercise is not an option, but a necessary, active, direct way that people can maintain good health, avoid illness, improve the quality of their lives, reduce their health care costs and extend their life expectancy.

Are You Investing In YOU? Asking The Right Questions

Below is a list of questions to help you identify how well you are investing in yourself, making daily deposits to your "human capital." You can use this tool to assess and reassess your "investment strategies" in you, as well as the potential progress you may be making with your Walking 4 Your Career & Finances program.

The questions below ask how frequently you practiced the following investments during the last month. Write down how often you practiced each by rating yourself (0 = Never, 1 = Almost Never, 2 = Sometimes, 3 = Fairly Often, 4 = Very Often).

Ask yourself, "In the last month, how often have I invested in myself by":

1. Walking or exercising regularly (At least four days per week).   _____

2. Eating healthy.   _____

3. Managing my stress.   _____

4. Sleeping at least seven to eight hours a day.   _____

5. Learning or studying something new and related to my field.   _____

6. Finding meaning and purpose in my work or interests.   _____

7. Meeting with my mentor, coach or network who help me in my work or interests.   _____

8. Volunteering to help others.   _____

9. Improving my people skills (e.g. public speaking or sales).   _____

10. Minimizing distractions and focusing on my work daily.   _____

Human Capital Investment This Month				
Very Low	Low	Average	High	Very High
0-10	11-20	20-29	29-34	35-40

If you scored very low, low or average this month you may want to consider implementing one or more of the following tips and techniques along with your Walking 4 Your Career & Finances program.

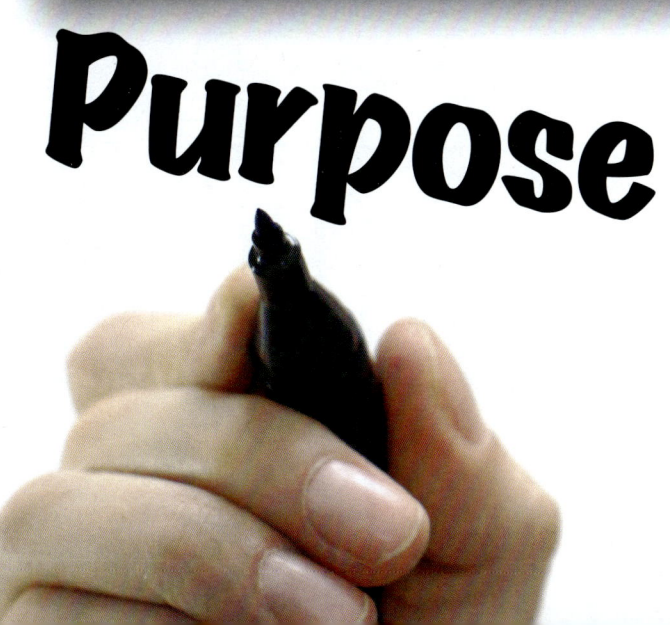

Purpose

Walking 4 Your Career & Finances

4 Ways To Boost Your Physical & Human Capital

If I were to pay you to exercise, how much would that influence your motivation to move on a regular basis? Health, business and human capital researchers have discovered a very powerful motivator for all of us to walk on a regular basis: Our "bottom line." Study after study points out that individuals who invest in their physical health boost their opportunities to make more today and in the future. Here are four proven and profitable strategies you can use to raise your "human capital" and future earning potential:

1 **Walk @ Work:** One of the best ways to get your walking in is to walk during nine to five. There are a number of strategies to help you do this— take a look at these tried and true methods:

   a   **Take the stairs:** Whenever possible make it a point to avoid the elevators and escalators when traveling or at work and take the stairs as much as possible. Every little bit counts!

   b   **Perform two-minute micro-walks:** Set your smart phone or a timer every hour to remind yourself to perform "chair walking" or to march in place. To perform "chair walking" while seated, move your feet and legs, hands and arms as if you were walking. This simple motion will increase your blood circulation, decrease stress and burn some extra calories. Even better, stand up march in place. It doesn't have to be long or in rhythm, just two minutes will do the trick! (See Cool Tools at the end of this chapter.)

   c   **Try to perform "micro burn interval walks":** Perform the "chair walking" or the march in place technique but this time move as fast as you can for 15 seconds, then walk slowly for 15 seconds. Repeat this for two to four minutes and you'll be boosting your energy and burning calories galore!

   d   **Have walk and talk meetings:** Take your weekly, seated office meeting outside and enjoy a "walk and talk" session with your group. Not only will it boost your personal health, fitness and human capital it will put a smile on everyone's face and raise those creative ideas to another level. This is also a great way to network and get to know one another better.

   e   **Explore treadmill desks:** Want to find a way to get your work done while you walk? Try a treadmill desk. Research over the last 10 years has shown sitting too long throughout your workday can wreak havoc on health and fitness. But using a treadmill desk is just one way you can move more throughout your busy day.

2 Build into your personal brand by investing in your education: Think of yourself as your own business—even if you are working for someone else. Ask yourself, "What would increase the value of my brand (me) for my present employer, clients, customers or colleagues?" Here are a few ways you can boost your brand, value and education while walking:

a Study for a certification, degree or graduate training: Using your smart phone or iPod download lectures and trainings related to your schooling, allowing you the opportunity to learn while you walk.

b Become well-rounded by listening to audio books: With so many great business, financial and health books in an audio version, you can become very well versed in a number of subjects while walking.

c Keep up on the trends in your industry: When walking, use your smart phone or iPod and listen to seminars or trend reports related to your field of work. You'll be in the know while you are on the go!

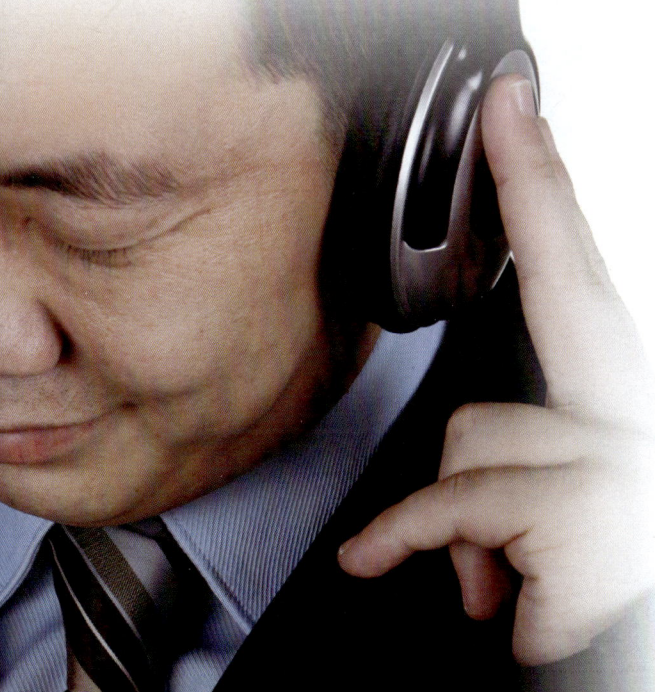

3 Get or become a mentor: One of the best investments you could ever make in your own or another's human capital is to consider the benefit of mentorship. Find someone you respect in your office or field of interest and ask them if they would meet with you for a "walk and talk" meeting on a regular basis. Let them know you'd love their input and help to become the best you can be in your career. Or build into someone else's career by walking and talking together with them weekly.

4 Practice, practice, practice: One of the best ways to boost your human capital is to become proficient and well versed in presenting. Whether it is to a small group, large audience or even a one-on-one conversation with a colleague, friend or family member, using your time when walking to practice your speech, pitch, idea or apology is a great way to improve your message, delivery and skills. Whether you are presenting an idea, service, product, opportunity or challenge, knowing what you want to say ahead of time and hearing yourself say it is a valuable skill you can use in every relationship you have.

Walk Well: Moving For Your Career Or Financial Future

Now that you've learned some proven human capital strategies to help with "Walking 4 Your Career & Finances," you are now ready to put it into practice. On the next page, you will find a "Capital Raising" routine that combines "micro walks" and "rolling" along with the mentioned human capital boosting techniques. If you'd prefer, you can also use one of the four walking styles in the previous "Body" or "Mind" chapters in conjunction with the strategies presented in this chapter. If you'd like a refresher on what type of walking is best for you go to pages 24 to 28. Be sure to select the type of walking routine you feel most confident you can accomplish and are physically ready to perform.

Walking 4 Your Career & Finances

Walking 4 Your Career & Finances: "Capital Walking Routine"

Goal—Increase your physical and human capital with this weekly walking routine.

- ✓ Take a two-minute Micro Walk @ Work every hour.
- ✓ Schedule your meetings as a "walk and talk."
- ✓ When walking, listen to lectures and audio books related to your industry or area of interest.
- ✓ Make it a point to walk with your mentor, coach or group weekly.
- ✓ Reassess your "Investments in YOU" weekly. See page 75 for questions.
- ✓ On a scale of 1-10, 1 = Easy, light breathing, 5 = Somewhat winded and 10 = Racing someone full speed, almost breathless, perform "Strolling" or "Rolling" at a two to five intensity and "Micro walks" or "Micro-Burning" can be performed anywhere from a two to seven intensity level.

Walking For Your Career & Finances: Capital Walking—Week 1 Goal: Five days per week. Focus on using "human capital" raising techniques this week, especially during your workday.

☀ DAY	🕐 WALKING WORKOUT	☰ INTENSITY
Monday	Micro-Walks—2 minutes every hour throughout your workday	2-6
Tuesday	Strolling—10 minutes during your workday	2-4
Wednesday	Micro-Walks—2 minutes every hour throughout your workday	2-6
Thursday	Strolling-Walk—10 minutes during your workday	2-4
Friday	Micro-Walks—2 minutes every hour throughout your workday	2-6
Saturday	Rest	
Sunday	Rest	

Your Next Steps—If you are ready, advance yourself to the next week recommendations:

Week 2: Your goal for week #2 is to complete five days of "Capital Walking", but this week perform three days of two to three minutes of "Micro-Burn Interval Walking," (every hour throughout your workday perform 15 seconds as fast as you can then 15 seconds slowly and repeat for two to three minutes) accumulating a total of 15-20 minutes on these days. On the two other days of the week increase your strolling to 15-20 minutes a day. This week, think about how you can "build into your personal brand", using your iPhone or iPod to boost your education and learning.

Week 3: Your goal for week #3 is to complete six days of "Capital Walking", but this week perform four days of two to four minutes of "Micro-Burn Interval Walking", (every hour throughout your workday, perform 15 seconds as fast as you can then 15 seconds slowly and repeat for two to four minutes) accumulating a total of 15-30 minutes on these days. On the three other days of the week increase your "strolling" to a "rolling" intensity and increase your time to 20-25 minutes a day. This week, focus on "Walking and Talking" with others in your company or neighborhood.

Week 4: Your goal for week #4 is to complete six days of "Capital Walking", but this week perform five days of three to four minutes of "Micro-Burn Interval Walking", (every hour throughout your workday, perform 15 seconds as fast as you can then 15 seconds slowly and repeat for three to four minutes) accumulating a total of 20-30 minutes on these days. On the other days of the week perform three days of "rolling" for 30 minutes before, during or after work. This week, focus on meeting with your mentor or becoming a mentor to someone you'd like to help.

Week 5 and beyond: Continue to perform Week #4 recommendations and utilize the various "human capital raising" techniques. Or choose one of the other Walking 4 Wellness plans found in Chapters 2, 3, 5 or 6.

*Remember, to avoid plateaus, it is very important to always challenge your body by walking faster, longer or more days.

Cool Tools

To help you boost your capital at work and combat sitting disease, check out these nifty walking tools:

1 Walking Desk: You can build movement throughout your workday by walking while you work using a "walking desk" or "treadmill desk." While moving at a comfortable pace throughout your day, you can lose weight, feel great and boost your capital all without breaking a sweat! Prices for "walking desks" can vary, but usually are between $400-$2,000. You can also create your own walking desk for under $50. You can upgrade your existing desk, with an additional

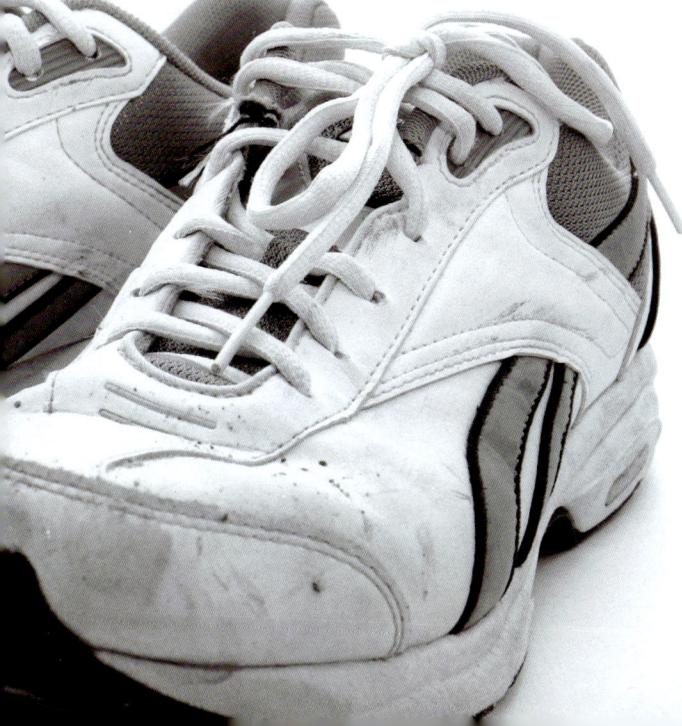

"lack" or "end" table, (check out your local office or furniture store, such as IKEA,) raising your computer screen and keyboard. Just remember that your keyboard should be at or slightly above elbow height, your monitor should maintain about a 20-degree upward tilt, and your eyes should stay about 24 to 28 inches from the screen. While standing during your day will require some getting used to, begin to walk or march in place while standing at various times during your day for a short period of time. If you own a treadmill you can use pre-made walking desks for under $500. Check out this site to start: **http://trekdesk.com/trekdesk**.

2 Voom: Voom is an online fitness program that is changing workers' workstations from the source of the problem to the solution. Voom prompts you to follow two-minute micro-break videos once an hour; a protocol developed using the latest research on inactivity physiology. In a fun, social online or smart phone format, Voom's goal is to provide you with the maximum benefits with the minimum amount of effort throughout your workday. You can go to **voomwell.com** to learn more or check out other programs and simple ideas designed to combat sitting disease, such as simply setting your smart phone alarm to go off every hour reminding you to get up from your desk and move.

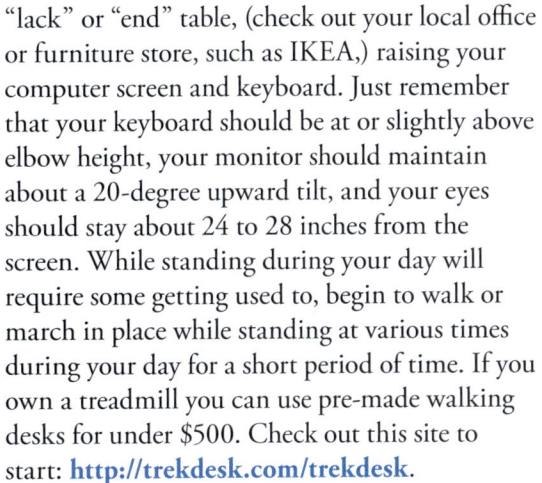

Chapter 5

Walking 4 Your Heart & Spirit

Simple Steps To Help You Walk With Purpose, Passion And Power

No road is long with good company.

TURKISH PROVERB

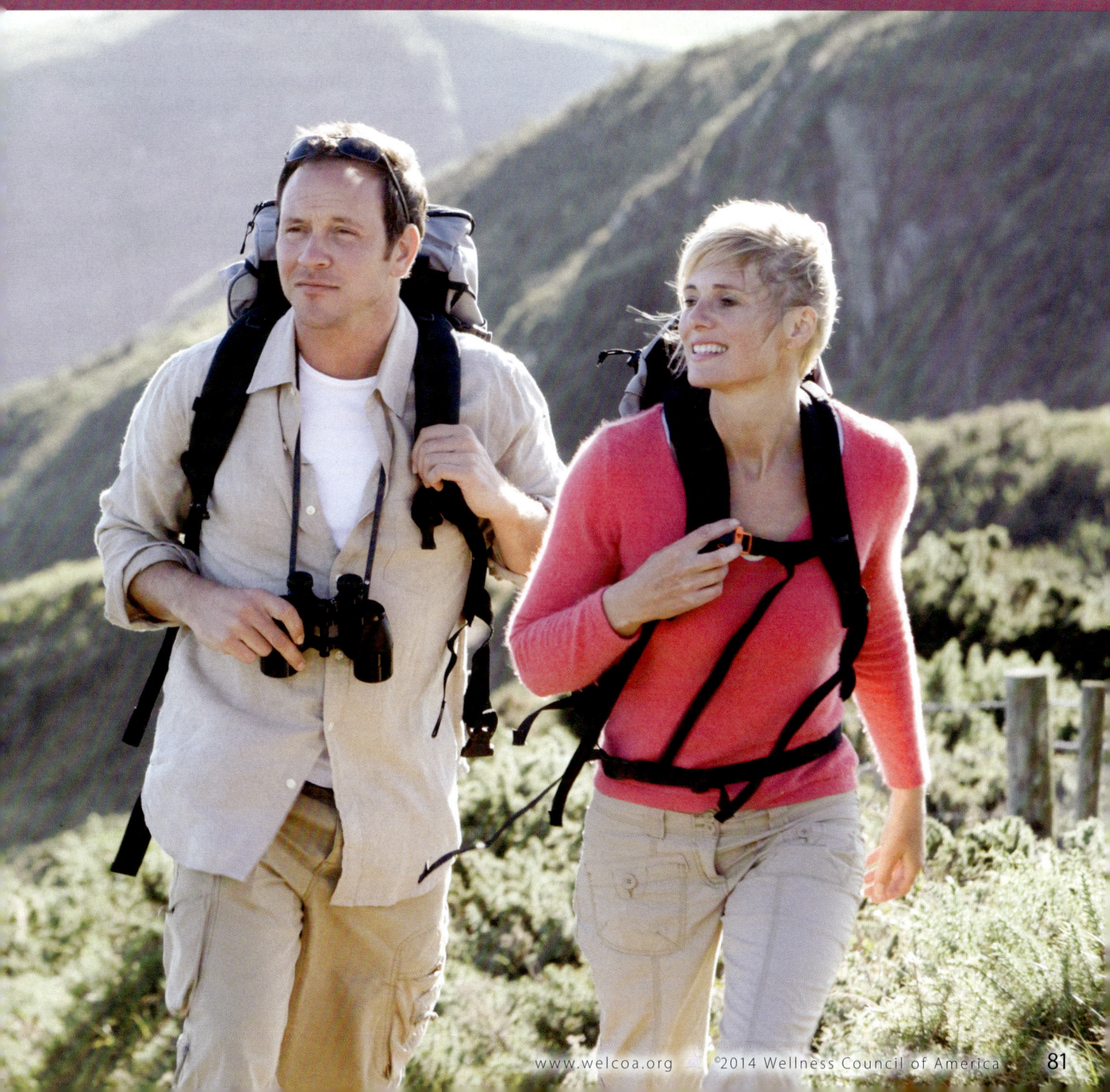

Walking 4 Your Heart & Spirit

Phone A Friend

Think of yourself on a game show. There is one question left. Answer it correctly and you win good health for the rest of your life. Answer it incorrectly and you'll have to go back to the beginning and learn from experience. Here's your last question: **According to the *Journal of Occupational and Environmental Medicine,* what factor influences our physical health the most?**

✓ Smoking

✓ Lack of exercise

✓ Poor nutrition

✓ Too much alcohol

✓ None of the above

Answer: None of the above.

According to scientific researchers, the source that influences our physical health more than anything else is not our diet. Not our exercise. Not how much we smoke. Or even how much stress we are under. It's how CONNECTED we are! The latest scientific research has found when we are disconnected from important life-giving sources that fill our heart and spirit, such as meaningful relationships and a sense of purpose and a passion for life, our attitudes, motivation to choose healthy behaviors and ultimately our health, suffer greatly. Are you skeptical? By the end of this chapter, you'll clearly see how walking for your heart and spirit can dramatically impact not only your relational, emotional and spiritual health, but it can also be one of the greatest motivators to help you get moving, stay moving and live well. In this chapter we will explore:

1 Why Walk 4 Your Heart And Spirit

2 Walking On Purpose—Larry's Story

3 The Greatest Motivator

4 Connecting To Your Heart And Spirit

5 Are You Connected? Asking The Right Questions

6 Four Ways To Connect To Your Heart & Spirit

7 Walk Well: Moving For Your Heart & Spirit

8 Cool Walking Tools

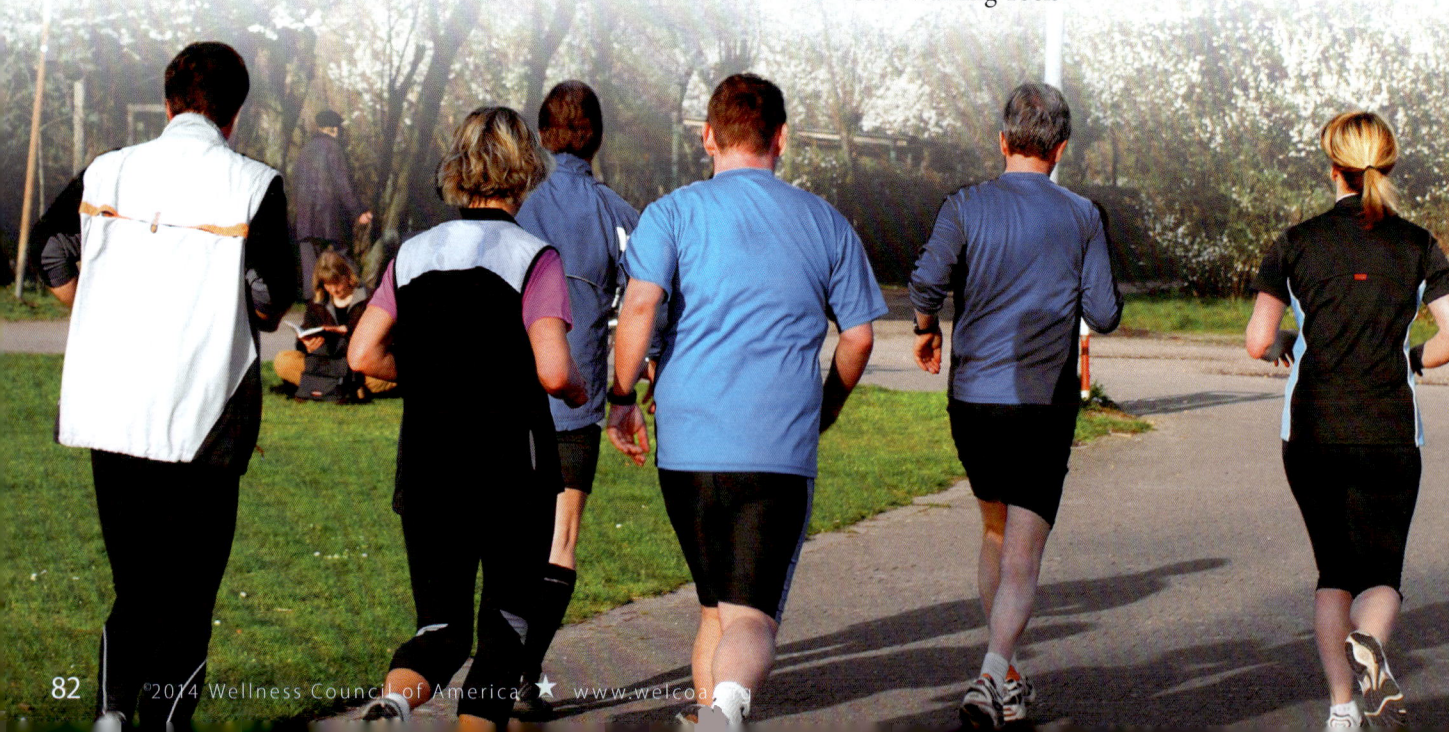

Why Walk 4 Your Heart And Spirit

According to the latest scientific research, individuals who walk for a cause and in community with others significantly increase their motivation and quality of their emotional, relational and spiritual health. Take a look at what the science says.

Regular walking for a cause and with others:

✓ Elevates your motivation to move more and to make better health decisions

✓ Increases social interaction

✓ Improves conversational skills

✓ Enhances marriage, intimacy, relationships, bonding and a sense of community

✓ Decreases feelings of loneliness, depression and despair

✓ Increases likelihood of starting and sticking with your walking routine

✓ Raises enthusiasm for life

✓ Boosts self-worth, attitude, meaning and purpose for life

✓ Increases longevity

✓ Speeds up recovery from injury and illness

✓ Elevates happiness and life satisfaction

✓ Improves the lives of others

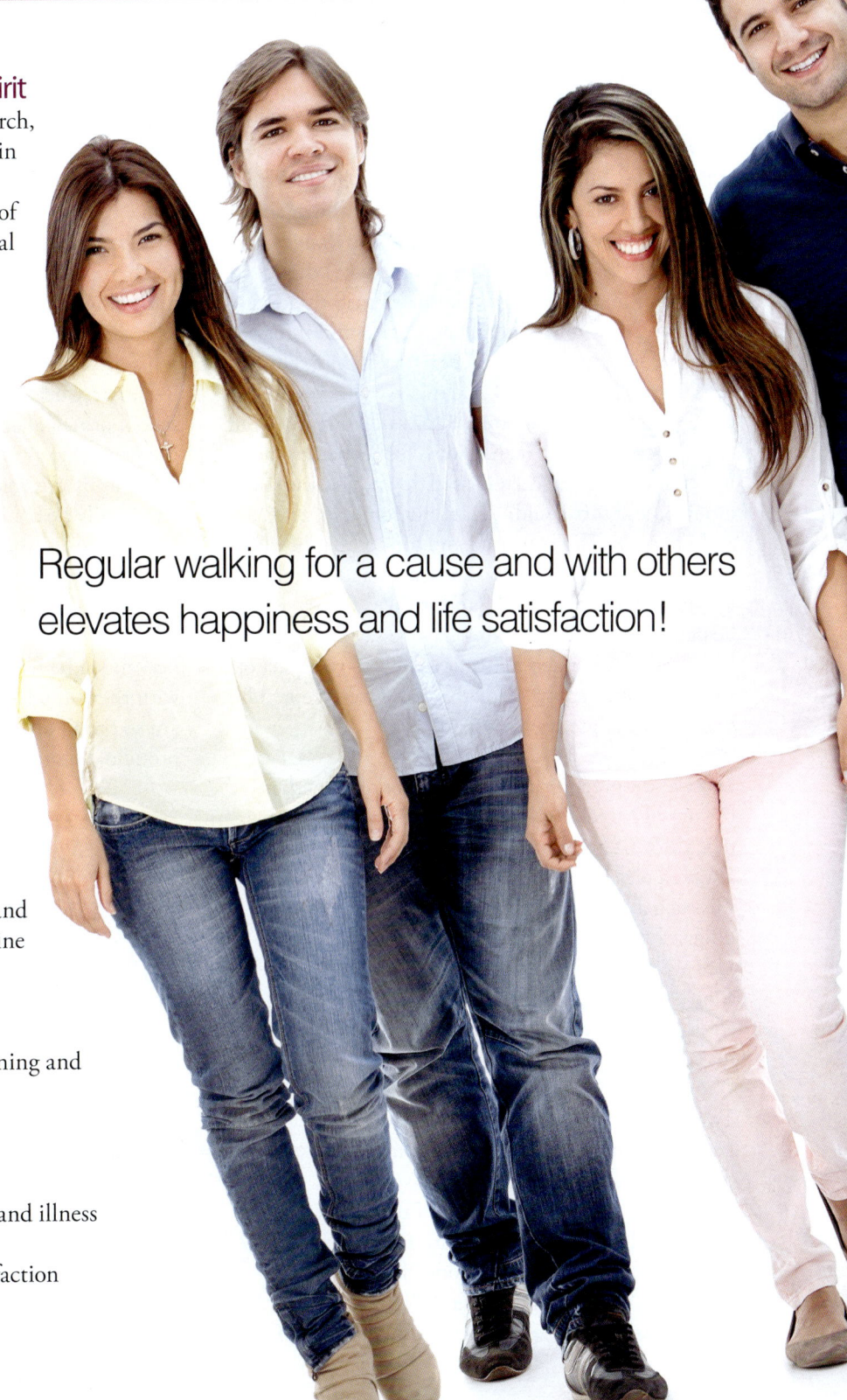

Regular walking for a cause and with others elevates happiness and life satisfaction!

Walking 4 Your Heart & Spirit

Walking On Purpose

Eight years ago, Larry was looking for a way to get fit and finally stay fit. Larry used to be a big time athlete but after years of neglecting his personal health and well-being he saw his weight skyrocket, fitness plummet and blood pressure and cholesterol rise to dangerous levels. I met Larry at a business conference where we were promoting a 12 Week Life Transformation program. Larry filled out an application and interviewed with me, hoping to be selected. After shaking hands and exchanging pleasantries, I asked Larry why he wanted to be a part of the program and he said, "I really want to get back in shape. Yeah, I want to feel better and look better, but…" Larry then looked down, pausing for a moment and softly said, "Sean, my son is 10 years old and I'm now 47." He paused and took a breath, then said, "My father passed away when I was 10," then looking up at me, he said, "and my dad was 47 when he passed away." Larry didn't have to say another word. I could see how much it meant to him to be a part of this program. He was ready to go and we accepted him unanimously into the program.

Larry and I grew very close as we worked together for the next 12 weeks, talking weekly by phone, as I was in California and Larry lived in South Dakota. It was always a pleasure to speak with him as he was such a kind and thoughtful man and diligently completed all I asked of him. Lifting weights, eating healthy and walking a lot, even in extremely cold South Dakota weather, Larry was determined to change his course.

Twelve weeks had flown by. It was time for Larry to fly back to California and reassess his progress. I remember like it was yesterday when I first saw him. The reason I remember is because I didn't recognize him. He walked up to me and said, "Sean!" I looked at the man standing in front of me and said, "Larry?" I was blown away! He looked 20 years younger and 40 pounds lighter. He was fit, strong, healthy and happy. Larry smiled and gave me a big bear hug. I have never seen a greater transformation in just 12 weeks. I asked Larry later what was the most important factor leading to his transformation. Larry said without hesitation, "With the love and help from my family, friends, fellow teachers, students and your weekly coaching, I have found my reason to move and keep on moving." Not only did Larry find his reason to move, he has made it his life's work and purpose to help transform others' lives. Larry decided to voluntarily leave his job as a high school principal and go back to the classroom teaching physical education to all of his students. Larry has now made it his mission to transform each and every student and family he comes into contact with and it's having a tremendous impact on his entire community. But most importantly to me is when I hear from Larry from time to time and how it warms my heart to hear how very proud he is of his now teenage son and daughter and how much he relishes each and every moment he has with them and his wife. Larry, you are an inspiration! I am so proud of you and I know your dad would be very proud of you too.

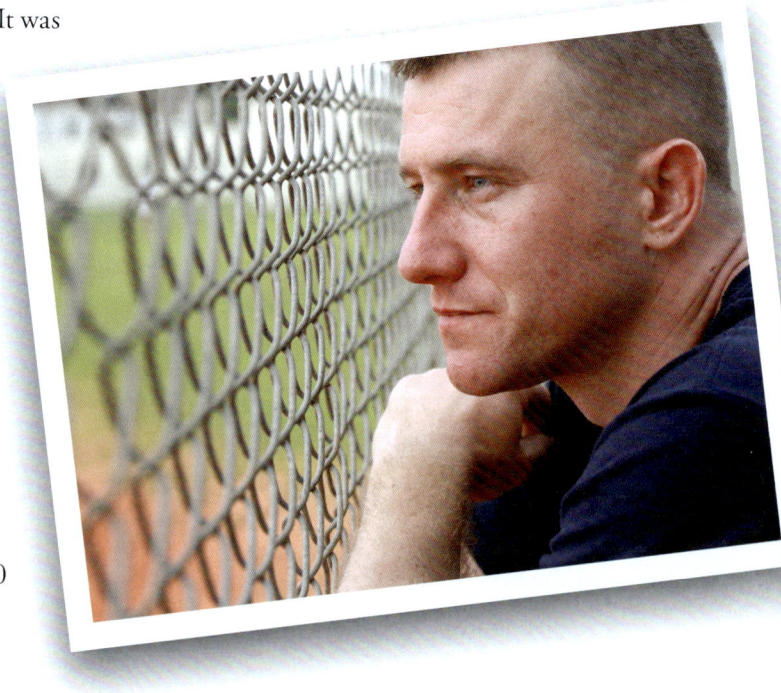

The Greatest Motivator

There have been a few major health studies in recent years that have significantly altered the way Americans care for our health. One breakthrough, in particular, was discovered by Dr. Dean Ornish, a Harvard trained physician who uncovered four proven steps to reverse (that's right, reverse) heart disease. All we have to do is:

1 Exercise regularly

2 Eat less fat and eat more veggies

3 Reduce stress

4 Quit smoking

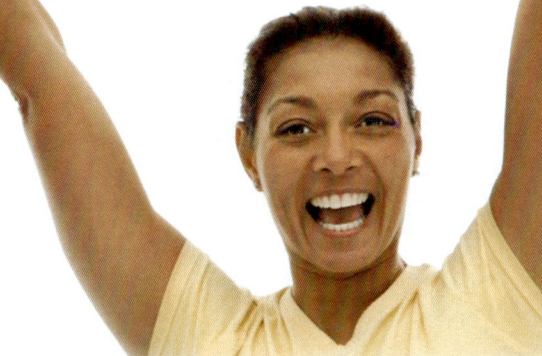

"People are much more likely to choose life-enhancing behaviors (like exercise and healthy eating) rather than self-destructive ones when they feel loved and cared for."

PSYCHOSOMATIC MEDICINE 4

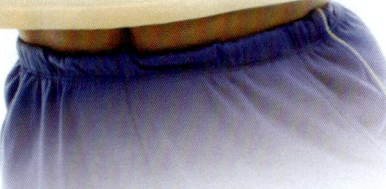

After his landmark work, a new bar was set for the medical community and you would think that Americans would have eagerly embraced and adopted Dr. Ornish's steps. But after a number of years of Americans going the other way, Dr. Ornish was left frustrated, defeated and perplexed. Why had so few followed his proven path to optimal health? So he began to search for answers. He realized just knowing what to do was only part of the solution. He asked, "What motivates an individual to live well?" After scouring hundreds of research articles and working with a team of researchers, Dr. Ornish came to a startling conclusion. Take a look at his synopsis:

"Medicine today seems to focus primarily on the physical and mechanistic: drugs and surgery, genes and germs, microbes and molecules. I am not aware of any other factor in medicine—not diet, not smoking, not exercise, not stress, not genetics, not drugs, not surgery—that has a greater impact on our quality of life, incidence of illness, and premature death from all causes than love and intimacy.

Love and intimacy are at the root of what makes us sick and what makes us well, what causes sadness and what brings us happiness, what makes us suffer and what leads to healing. If a new drug had the same impact, virtually every doctor in the country would be recommending it for his or her patients."

Let that sit for a bit. Read that last paragraph again. Dr. Ornish and other leading researchers have scoured years of data, all leading to the reality of "anything that affects your emotional, relational or spiritual health (i.e. affecting your experience of loving or being loved), can significantly impact your physical well-being—positively or negatively."

In other words, when we are CONNECTED—experiencing love, nurturing, acceptance, meaning, purpose, being cared for and supported—we are much more likely to be happier and healthier.

Walking 4 Your Heart & Spirit

Connecting To Your Heart And Spirit

Can love and community help heal what drugs, diets, fitness plans, doctors and surgeries alone can't heal? The latest research and scientific evidence confirms that well-connected human relationships are "one of the main missing links" to thriving emotional and physical health. The latest research also demonstrates that individuals who have a "strong internal or intrinsic spiritual practice or faith" and CONNECT to it regularly have significantly better mental and physical health than those who don't identify as having a meaningful spiritual practice or faith.

Researchers from Harvard, Duke and Yale universities have been conducting and analyzing more than 1,500 research studies on the impact community, spiritual practices and faith have upon health. Overwhelmingly, these studies demonstrate that people who CONNECT in a faith-based community regularly and consistently have less heart disease, fewer strokes, lower blood pressure, less depression, faster recovery from illness…and may even live longer.

A number of recent studies have found a significant relationship between a CONNECTEDNESS to having a cause or faith community and longer survival. A research study published in the *Annals of Behavioral Medicine* found that people who CONNECTED regularly to their spiritual practice, faith and place of worship were more likely to become physically active, to quit smoking, be less depressed, increase social relationships and initiate and maintain stable marriages. Conversely, research studies have found that a lack of CONNECTEDNESS to community, a spiritual practice or faith involvement can have a significant negative effect on a person's health.

We are happiest and most successful when we are in touch with ourselves, our friends, family, our community, our purpose, our cause and our faith.

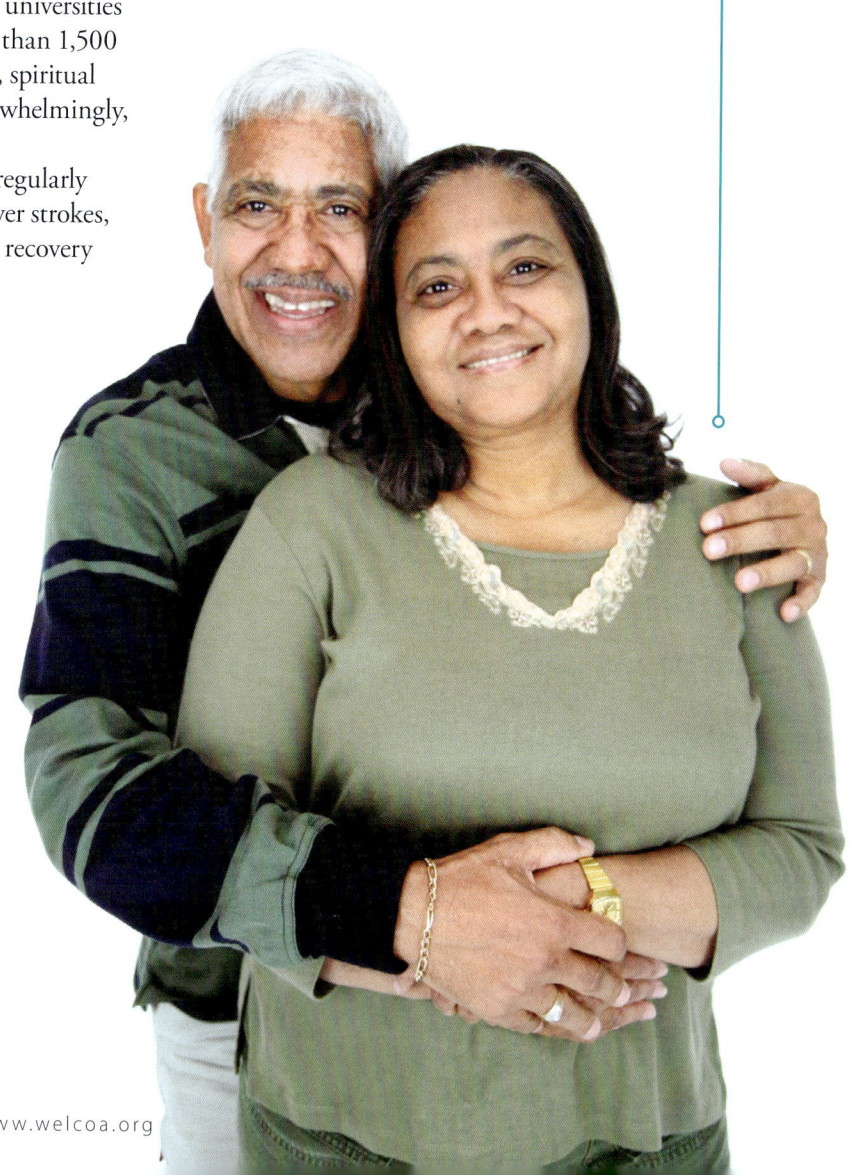

For example, when we are not connected, research demonstrates that:

1 The likelihood of engaging in unhealthy coping behaviors such as smoking, drinking in excess and overeating increases

2 The likelihood that we will make healthy lifestyle choices that are life enhancing rather than self-destructive decreases

3 The likelihood of premature disease and death from all causes increases by 200-500% or more

4 We are kept from fully experiencing the joy of everyday life

Additionally, according to the results of more than 78 research studies, Dr. David Larson, psychiatrist and president of the National Institute for Healthcare Research, (NIHR) and colleagues determined in the majority of cases a spiritual practice or meaningful faith can significantly enhance physical health.

Bottom line: We are happiest and most successful when we are in touch with ourselves, our friends, family, our community, our purpose, our cause and our faith. When we are connected, we feel hopeful, empowered and supported. We make positive choices that are beneficial for ourselves and helpful for others. Learning to nurture yourself, developing positive, helpful relationships, and pursuing your spiritual practice or faith are extremely important in sustaining an active, healthy, physically fit life.

Are You Connected? Asking The Right Questions

Below is a list of questions to help you identify how well you are connecting to your meaningful relationships, spiritual practice or faith. You can use this tool to assess and reassess any progress you may be making with your Walking 4 Your Heart & Spirit program. The questions below ask you how frequently you practiced the following during the last month. Write down how often you practiced each by rating yourself (0 = Never, 1 = Almost Never, 2 = Sometimes, 3 = Fairly Often and 4 = Very Often).

Ask yourself, "In the last month, how often have I invested in my heart or spirit by":

1. Intentionally connecting with those closest to me. (e.g. date night, letter, phone call). _____

2. Listening with an open mind and communicating effectively. _____

3. Finding ways to have fun, laugh and enjoy those closest to me. _____

4. Resolving any conflict in a positive way. _____

5. Sharing my heart with those closest to me. _____

6. Asking forgiveness when I have wronged others. _____

7. Forgiving others when I have been wronged. _____

8. Meeting regularly in a healthy community (e.g. church, synagogue, support group). _____

9. Being generous with my time. _____

10. Making a difference in the lives of others. _____

Heart & Spirit Health This Month				
Very Low	Low	Average	High	Very High
0-10	11-20	20-29	29-34	35-40

If you scored very low, low, or average this month you may want to consider implementing one or more of the following tips and techniques along with your Walking 4 Your Heart & Spirit program.

Walking strengthens the body, rejuvenates the mind and enlivens the spirit.

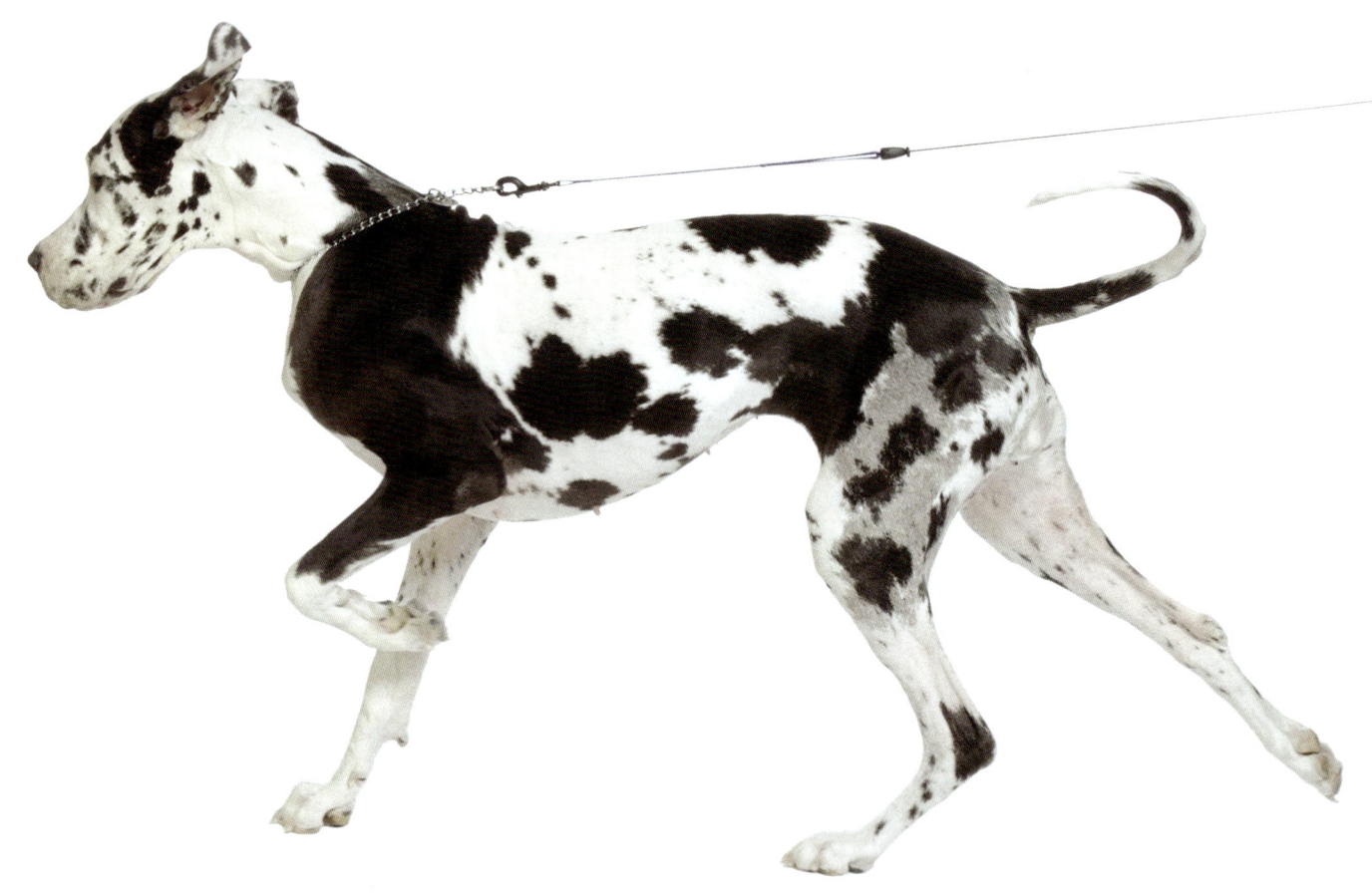

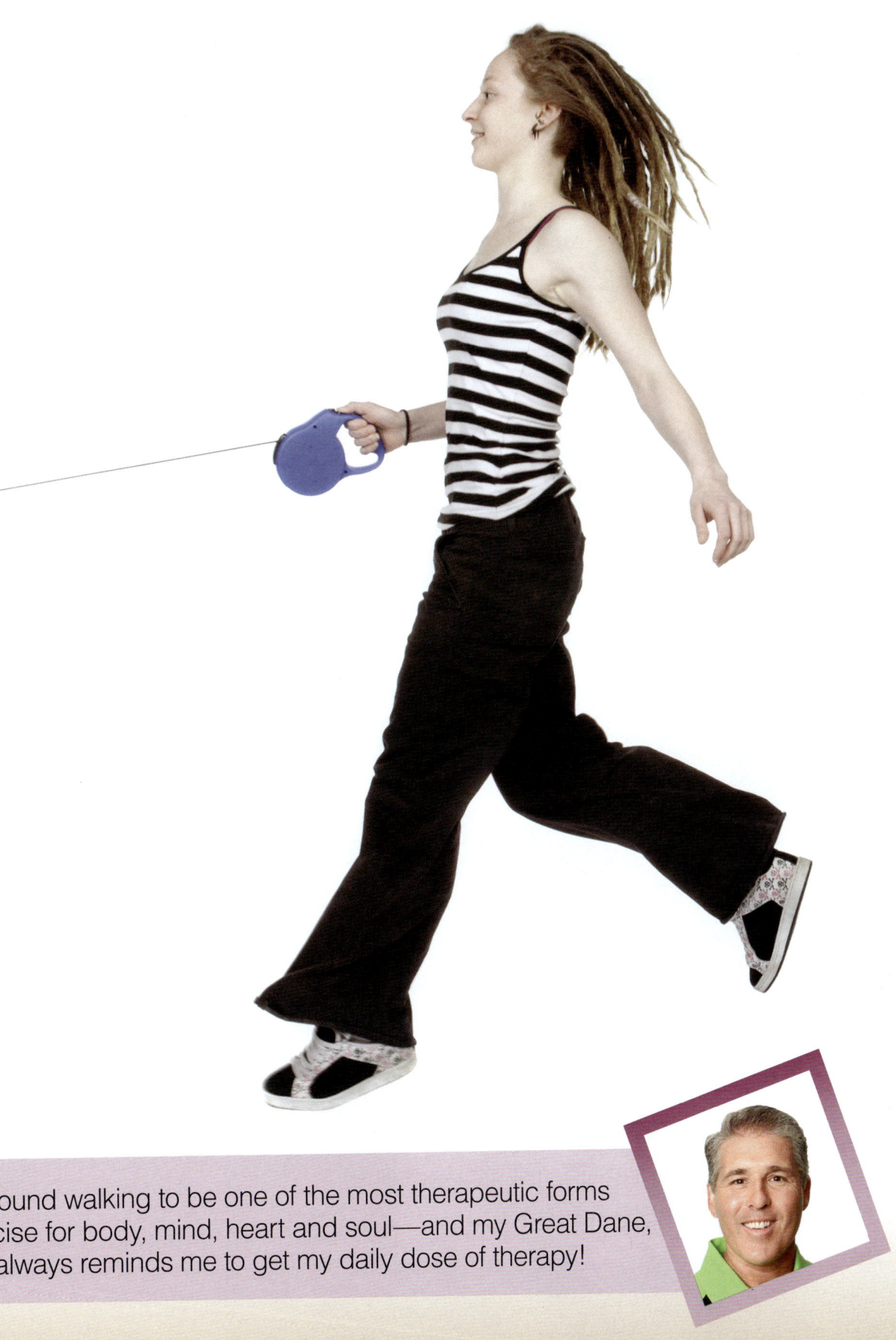

I have found walking to be one of the most therapeutic forms of exercise for body, mind, heart and soul—and my Great Dane, Sadie, always reminds me to get my daily dose of therapy!

Walking 4 Your Heart & Spirit

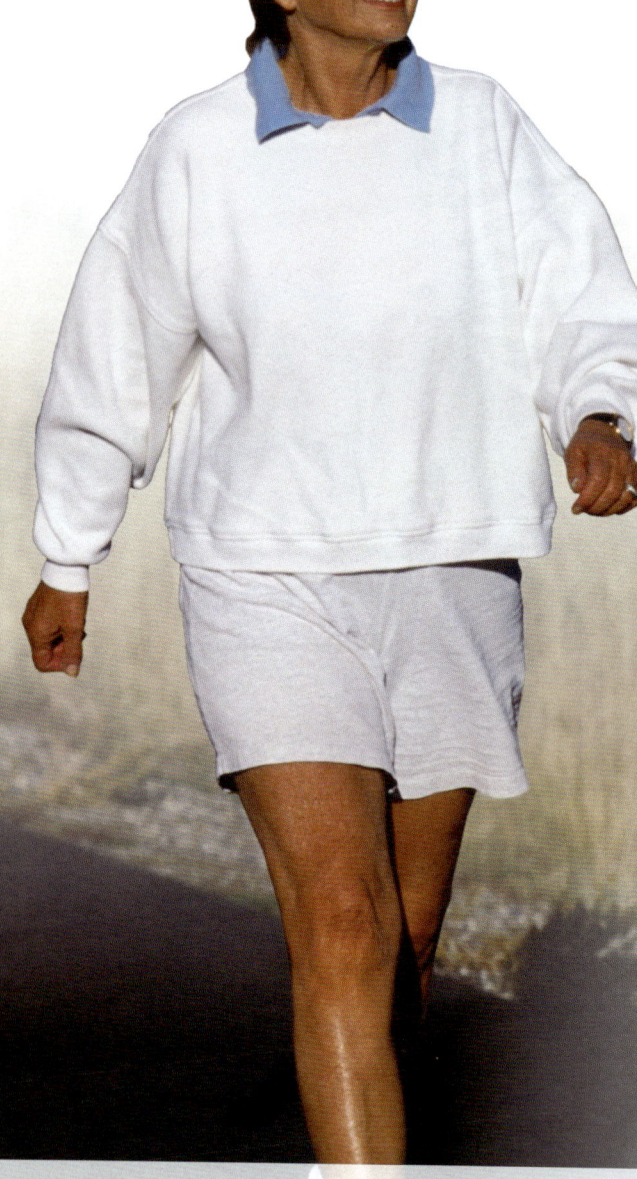

> When we have support, life is much more meaningful, richer, happier and altogether better.

Four Ways To Connect To Your Heart & Spirit

Philosophers, counselors, theologians and healers of various backgrounds for centuries understood when the heart and spirit were not well—the body was not well. Conversely, when the heart and spirit are well—the body is well. Recent research confirms this ancient thinking and has drawn the same conclusion; individuals who connect to their heart and spirit regularly enhance their physical health dramatically.

Here are four proven practices you can use to fill your heart and spirit before, during or after your walk:

1   Walk And Share Your Heart With A Buddy:
Studies show our lives thrive when we are deeply connected to our family, friends and community. When we have support, life is much more meaningful, richer, happier and altogether better. Fitness is no different. The science is in; the best way to ensure your fitness success is to combine fitness with friends. Here's a proven strategy to help you share your heart with those you care about:

Try sharing your "highs/victories" and "lows/challenges" for the day or week when walking. One of the best ways to share what's going on in your life with your buddy is to begin by sharing what is going well and not so well in your life. Begin by sharing what you are most grateful and thankful for with your friend. These would be considered your victories or highs for the day or week. Then have your buddy do the same. Sharing what you are excited, happy or thankful for and hearing the same from your buddy is a great way to remind yourself of the many blessings you both have. You'll both feel better after sharing what's going well. Next, share what you may be frustrated with, or the "low" point or "challenge" of your day or week. And have your friend do the same. Sharing your challenges or lows of the day or week to a sensitive caring buddy may be the best medicine to heal an empty or hurting heart.

2   **You've Got The Touch:** Touch is good for our health. When we receive a friendly, comforting hug, pat on the back or meaningful touch, our bodies release oxytocin, also known as "the love hormone" which has been found to decrease stress, lower blood pressure, reduce pain and help us feel good. For years, many respected psychologists and relationship experts would agree with the following recommendation: "We need four hugs a day for survival. We need eight hugs a day for maintenance. We need 12 hugs a day for growth." Regardless of the recommendation, according to researchers, the more hugs you get, the healthier you'll be. Hugging is one of the best ways to heal sickness, disease, loneliness, depression, anxiety and stress. Here are a few ways to get in your hugs as well as some other healing and comforting ways to touch and fill your heart and spirit before, during or after your walk:

a   **Hug Yourself**—If you don't have someone near you to hug, believe it or not, researchers at the University of Texas discovered "self-hugging"—wrapping your arms around yourself and squeezing actually releases oxytocin and other feel good biochemicals reducing pain and also boosting your health and well-being. Try giving yourself a hug before, during or after your walk—that's three hugs down and nine more to go!

b   **Hold Hands**—Studies show the simple caring act of holding your loved one's hand helps to reduce stress and enhance your relationship. Give it a try. Next time you are walking with a loved one, grab their hand on your stroll. Not only will you be the cutest couple in the neighborhood, but you will also be enhancing your physical, relational and mental health.

c   **Give And Get A Massage**—The simple act of rubbing your loved one's shoulders and visa versa is one of the best things you can do after a long walk or for that matter any time of day. Rubbing one's shoulders is a sign of affection and care as well as a great way to increase blood circulation and reduce stress, muscle tension, and aches and pains.

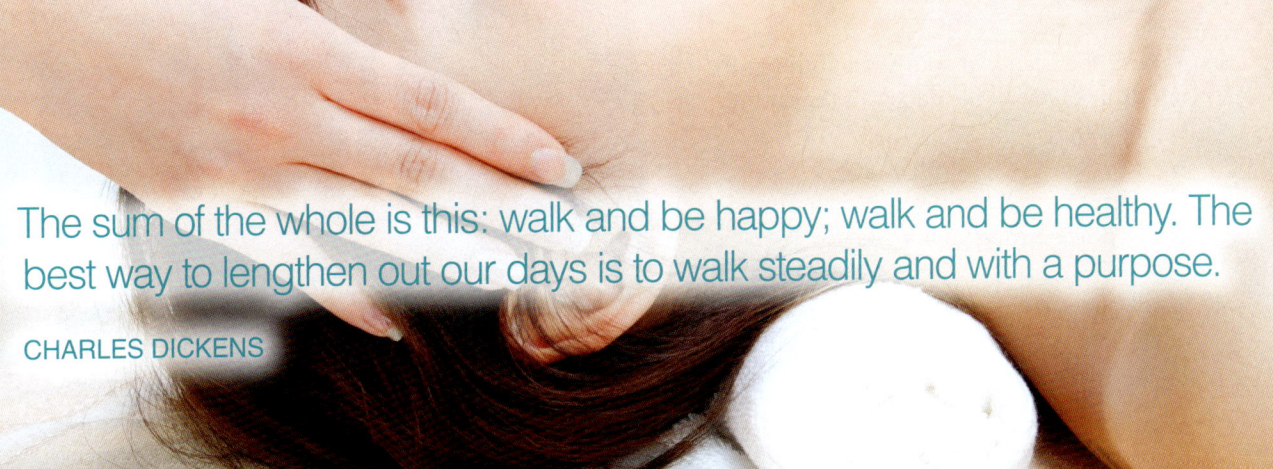

The sum of the whole is this: walk and be happy; walk and be healthy. The best way to lengthen out our days is to walk steadily and with a purpose.

CHARLES DICKENS

Walking 4 Your Heart & Spirit

3 **Cultivate Your Spirituality When You Walk:**
Over the centuries, the simple act of walking has played an enormous role in the devotional and spiritual lives of individuals all over the world. From pilgrimages to sacred sites to walking the dog around the block, these daily rituals are designed to ease our burdens, boost our spirit, and provide comfort, peace, hope and faith to our frequently busy and stress filled lives. Try one of the following exercises for your heart and spirit the next time you lace up your walking shoes:

✓ At the beginning or during your walk, think about all the things in your life you are most thankful for. If walking with a buddy, share them with each other.

✓ Sing or listen to your favorite song while walking. Find music that is devotional, worshipful, inspirational or upbeat—something that fills your heart and spirit and boosts your faith and hope.

✓ Meditate when you walk—pay close attention to your breathing, taking pleasure in each breath. Or count your footsteps, counting "one, two, one, two" or recite a sacred prayer or scripture repetitively.

✓ Pray during your walk. Nothing fancy needed. Be honest about where you are and what's going on in your heart.

✓ Take in the beauty of your surroundings. Be mindful. Enjoy all the details of the nature before you.

✓ Visualize yourself healthy, happy, balanced and at peace during your walk.

✓ Think about taking a walk to someone's home or work and perform a random act of kindness.

✓ When walking, make eye contact and focus on smiling when you encounter others. You'll most likely get a smile back, which fills their heart and yours.

✓ If you are walking with a buddy or group, take some time to share a quality or strength you really like in each other.

✓ After your walk is over, find a place of rest and sit silently for a few minutes—perform deep breathing if you would like as well.

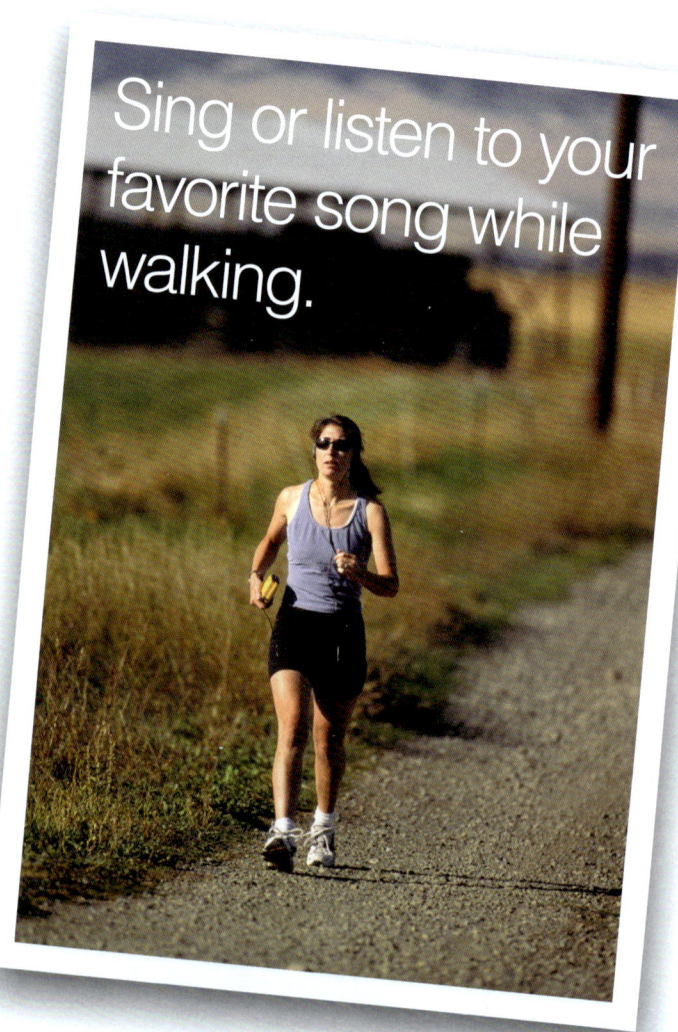

Sing or listen to your favorite song while walking.

4 Walk On Purpose—Find Your Cause:

Walking for charity or for a cause is one of the best things you can do for your body, heart and spirit. Knowing that you are helping another or a caring organization, and easing the pain or difficulty of others through your efforts is deeply spiritual and fills our hearts. It's also a great motivator to help get and stay fit.

Charity walks vary from just a mile to going on for days or even weeks. Some charity walks/runs encourage you to dress up in your favorite costume or get doused with different colors or take you through difficult terrain. Take a look at the list below and consider signing up for a walking cause that touches your heart and spirit.

▶ AIDS Walk
  aidswalk.net

▶ American Diabetes Association
  stepout.diabetes.org

▶ Alzheimer's Association Memory Walk
  alz.org/memorywalk

▶ Arthritis Walk: Let's Move Together Arthritis Foundation
  letsmovetogether.org

▶ Breast Cancer 3-Day: Susan G. Komen For The Cure
  the3day.org

▶ Buddy Walk: National Down Syndrome Society
  buddywalk.org

▶ Charity Miles App: Use this app to track your walking miles on your mobile device and earn money for charities!
  charitymiles.org

▶ Avon Walk For Breast Cancer
  avonwalk.org

▶ Drunk Driving: Walk Like MADD
  walklikemadd.org

▶ Heart Disease: Start!
  Heart Walk: American Heart Association
  startwalkingnow.org/start_heart_walk.jsp

▶ Hunger: World Food Programme
  wfp.org/content/walk-the-world

▶ Idita Walk
  idita-walk.com

▶ NAMI Walks: National Alliance Of Mental Illness
  namiwalks.org

▶ Relay For Life: American Cancer Society
  relayforlife.org

▶ Walk For Wishes: Make A Wish Foundation Of America
  wish.org/news/events

Walk Well: Moving For Your Heart And Spirit

Now that you've learned some proven strategies to help with "Walking 4 Your Heart & Spirit," you are now ready to put it into practice. On the next page, you will find a "Heart & Spirit" routine focusing on meditative "strolling" and "hiking" along with the mentioned relational and spiritual boosting techniques. If you'd prefer, you can also use one of the four walking styles in the previous "Body," "Mind," or "Career & Finances" chapters in conjunction with the strategies presented in this chapter. If you'd like a refresher on what type of walking is best for you go to pages 24 to 28. Be sure to select the type of walking routine you feel most confident you can accomplish and are physically ready to perform.

Walking 4 Your Heart & Spirit

Walking 4 Your Heart & Spirit Routine

Goal—Increase your relational and spiritual health with this weekly walking routine.

- ✓ Walk and share your heart with a buddy.

- ✓ Get and give meaningful touch; hugs, self-hugs, hand holding, massage.

- ✓ Cultivate your spirituality; be thankful, meditate, pray, sing and take in the beauty of your surroundings.

- ✓ Walk on purpose—find your cause.

- ✓ Reassess your "Heart and Spirit health" weekly. See page 87 for questions.

- ✓ On a scale of 1-10, 1 = Easy, light breathing, 5 = Somewhat winded and 10 = Racing someone full speed, almost breathless, perform "Strolling" at a two to five intensity.

Walking For Your Heart & Spirit—Week 1 Goal: Six days per week. Focus on using the recommended "Heart & Spirit" techniques this week.

☀ DAY	🕐 WALKING WORKOUT	≣ INTENSITY
Monday	Strolling—20 minutes	2-5
Tuesday	Strolling—20 minutes	2-5
Wednesday	Strolling—20 minutes	2-5
Thursday	Strolling—20 minutes	2-5
Friday	Strolling—20 minutes	2-5
Saturday	Strolling/Hike—45 minutes in nature	2-5
Sunday	Rest	

Your Next Steps—If you are ready, advance yourself to the next week recommendations:

Week 2: Your goal for week #2 is to complete six days of "Heart and Spirit" walking, but this week perform 30 minutes of "strolling" everyday except Saturday. This Saturday, increase to a 60-minute hike or nature walk. This week, ask your spouse, child, family member or a close friend to walk with you and share your "high's" and "lows" for the day or week. If you feel comfortable, also try and use touch as part of your walk—holding hands, using massage or hugs before and after your walk.

Week 3: Your goal for week #3 is to complete six days of "Heart and Spirit" walking, but this week perform 45 minutes of "strolling" everyday except Saturday. This Saturday, increase to a 75-minute hike or nature walk. This week, focus on cultivating your spirituality before, during and after your walk. See page 92 for ideas.

Week 4: Your goal for week #4 is to complete six days of "Heart and Spirit" walking, but this week perform 45-60 minutes of "strolling" everyday except Saturday. This Saturday, increase to a 90-minute hike or nature walk. This week, take some time to consider walking for a cause. If this isn't something you'd like to do right now, consider what is your motivation and reason to walk.

Week 5 and beyond: Continue to perform week #4 recommendations and utilize the various "Heart & Spirit" techniques. Or choose one of the other Walking 4 Wellness plans found in Chapters 2, 3, and 4.

*Remember, to avoid plateaus, it is very important to always challenge your body by walking faster, longer or more days.

Cool Walking Tools

To help you invest in your heart and spirit, check out these cool walking tools:

1 Activity Trackers: From waist wearing pedometers to fashionable colored bracelet bands, movement trackers are fast becoming very popular tools to measure not only your walking but also areas such as sleep, nutrition and activity throughout your day. Products such as Jawbone UP, Fitbit Flex and Nike+ Fuel Band are just a few of the latest motion bands which sync or connect your daily stats to your smart phone or computer, allowing you to track your number of steps, active minutes, calories expended, sleep and distance covered. Several apps also provide food intake and mood throughout the day and also provide additional tools, information and motivation to help you reach your personal goals. Prices and features vary so be sure to try out as many as you can before purchasing.

You may also want to check out websites such as **www.consumerreports.org** to learn more before making an investment.

2 The Daniel Plan: is a comprehensive faith-based wellness program integrating faith, food, fitness, focus and friends. With best selling authors, Rick Warren, Dr. Daniel Amen and Dr. Mark Hyman, this book promises to fill the hearts and spirits of your church, synagogue, company or organization.

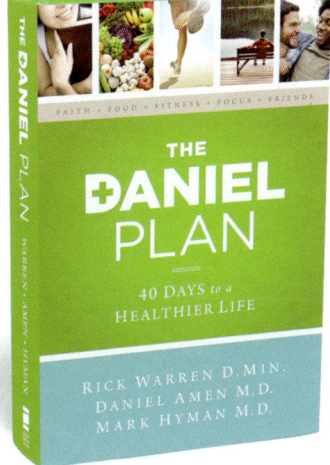

Chapter 6

Walking 4 Living Well

Simple steps to help you get moving and keep moving!

To me, if life boils down to one thing, it's movement.
To live is to keep moving."

JERRY SEINFELD

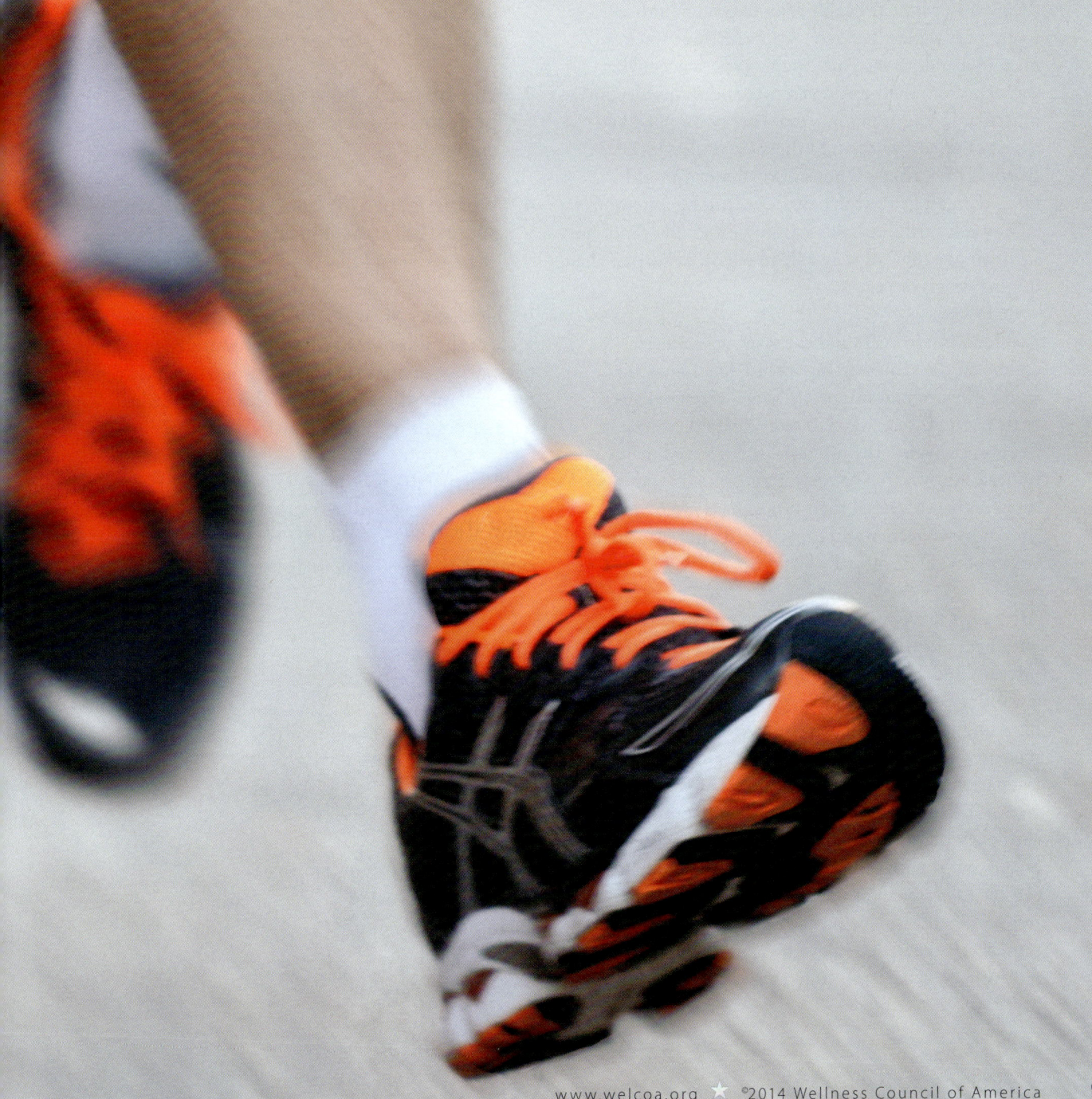

Walking 4
Living Well

In 1966, five 20-year-old men assembled in the Southwestern Medical Center in Dallas, Texas to assist NASA scientists in understanding the impact of weightlessness and inactivity in space travel. To begin the study, all five participants were to complete a battery of physiological tests to evaluate their cardiovascular health prior to going on three weeks of complete bed rest. After the three weeks of no activity, all of the participants experienced what was expected, their cardiovascular endurance declined, muscular strength plummeted, energy dropped and a host of other health and fitness issues developed. **Bottom line, they all got out of shape and old fast.** Then all five participants were put on a rigorous eight-week cardiovascular training program—and, not surprisingly, they all were able to regain or surpass their original levels of fitness.

Fast forward 30 years and the same researchers contacted the same participants to do a follow up study. The original five participants were now 50-51 years old and were asked to re-evaluate their fitness levels once again. The five now middle-aged men underwent the same battery of assessments and shockingly discovered their fitness levels were now similar to what they had experienced after just three weeks of bed rest 30 years ago.

After their testing, the five participants were then put on a tailored exercise program based upon their interests and what they enjoyed. Two of the men began a walking program, two a jogging program and one a bicycling program. All exercise levels were gradually increased to the original testing levels in the 1966 evaluation, roughly four to five hours of exercise a week. Then after six months of exercise training, their cardiovascular fitness and endurance was reassessed. Surprisingly, with only a few months of moderate aerobic exercise, all of the now middle-aged men had restored their aerobic and cardiovascular fitness to the same levels they once enjoyed when they were 20 years old! What can we learn from this?

1　**Inactivity ages you faster than anything else.** Just three weeks of bed rest led to 30 years of physiological aging!

2　**You can reverse decades of physiological aging and improve multiple areas of your life** with moderate exercise such as walking consistently performed over just a few months!

3　**You are much more apt to consistently perform** an exercise program you enjoy versus one you do not.

4　**We can learn a lot from those who have successfully traveled ahead of us**—helping us to get fit and stay fit.

In this chapter, we will review and introduce you to some of the most powerful and proven steps, tips and tricks you can use to help you get moving and keep moving. You will learn firsthand from individuals who have successfully learned how to Walk 4 Wellness!

Got grandkids? Throw on your shoes and take them on a walk! It's a great way to connect and build dialogue.

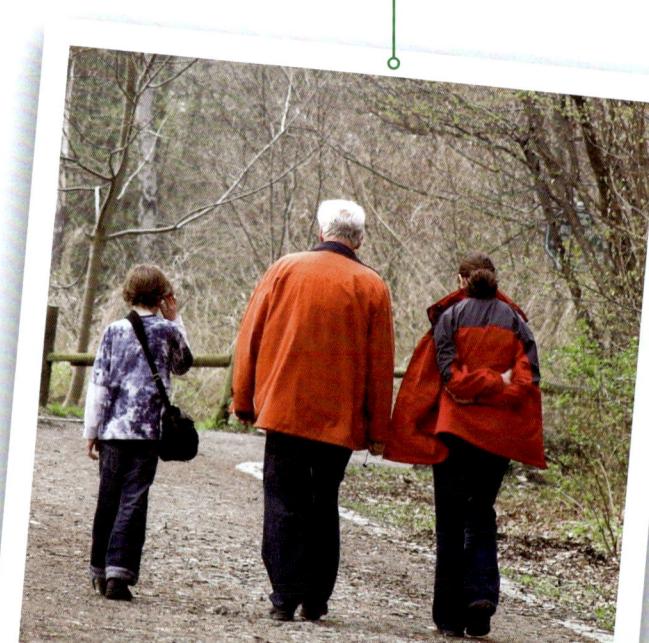

1 Think Of One Small "Win" Every Day

"My number one tip to help others get moving is to 'think of one small win' you can achieve every day. I took this idea and 'ran' with it. Actually I 'walked' with it! I decided I was going to start walking to get back in shape and began with walking for just a few minutes a day. That's it! I made it my 'win' to walk one or two more minutes each day I went for a walk. That was years ago! I'm now up to walking for an hour and a half a day almost every other day and I am at my high school weight again and I've never felt better!"

—Liz, 45, Mom

Liz found her victory in setting small, doable "wins" or steps every day. You can too! By choosing to focus on small "wins" every day—little steps you know you can accomplish, such as:

- ✓ Walk a 100 more steps today than you did yesterday

- ✓ Walk one more minute than you did yesterday

- ✓ Take one more flight of stairs today than you did yesterday

With this approach, you will find your confidence and fitness soaring to new levels.

> By choosing to focus on small "wins" every day—little steps you know you can accomplish, you will find your confidence and fitness soaring to new levels.

2 Take A Breath

"I've learned to carve out time in my day for myself. It was hard at first. I guess I didn't realize how valuable I was. After having heart surgery, I do now! I've learned to schedule time for myself every day to go for a walk to unwind and just take a break for myself. Some days I walk longer than others. But every day I make it a point to carve out, what I like to call my "breathing room," where I can take time to recharge my batteries and take care of me."

—Jim, 52, Software Manager

Flight attendants tell us when we are just about to take off: "If we experience unexpected turbulence and your oxygen mask deploys, when traveling with a child, please place the mask on yourself first before assisting your child." This is good advice and something many of our Walking 4 Wellness clients have learned. In order for us to help others and be our best, we need to take time to renew and recharge our batteries every day. So take Jim's advice, be intentional with your Walking 4 Wellness by:

- ✓ Scheduling your walking before the week begins

  - Use your smart phone to schedule days and times you are selecting to go for your walk

- ✓ Set up a "Gone Walking" sign on your office or kitchen door

- ✓ Schedule your alarm on your smart phone to remind you to take a breather and go for a walk

- ✓ Ask a family member or close friend to ask you weekly if you are investing in yourself and taking time for you

Walking 4 Living Well

3 Give Yourself A Break

"I have always been my worst critic. When I wouldn't lose weight every week or I ate too much or missed a workout, I'd find myself going into a spiral and losing motivation to be healthy altogether. I'd just throw my hands up in the air and quit. One day a close friend of mine told me I would do much better with my health and fitness goals if I were to give myself a break. He was right! As soon as I started focusing on what I could control and let go of what I couldn't and stopped beating myself up, I actually began to see my health and fitness improve. I'd tell everyone who is thinking about getting fit or staying fit, you've got to learn to give yourself a break. Nobody is perfect."

—Bruce, 53, Executive

It's true. Individuals who live healthy and fit lives are not perfect. They don't eat perfectly. They don't exercise perfectly. They have good days and bad days. What they do differently is they have found a way to learn from their challenges and consistently continue to do the things they know are best for their health and well-being. Simply put, unrealistic expectations or all-or-nothing thinking can lead to feeling guilty, beating yourself up and ultimately an excuse to quit and stop walking altogether. Just remember you don't have to be perfect to be fit!

4 Get A Buddy

"I learned early on, having a buddy, someone who would take the time to walk with me was one of the best things I could do for my health and fitness. When I don't feel like going, my friends remind me how good I'll feel if I just do it. That's all I need, a reminder to take care of myself!"

—Bev, 42, Human Resource Consultant

Bev found what studies show. Our lives thrive when we are deeply connected to our family, friends and community. When we have support, life is much more meaningful, richer, happier and altogether better. Fitness is no different. The science is in; the best way to ensure your fitness success is to combine fitness with friends. Here are a few ways you can strengthen your step with the power of friendship and fitness:

- ✓ Walk with a family member (spouse, child or loved one)

- ✓ Join a walking or hiking group

- ✓ Get a dog

- ✓ Share your fitness schedule and progress daily or weekly via Twitter, Facebook or other social media outlets

5 Motion = Emotion

"The best thing about walking for me is how happy it makes me feel! Every day I am pulled in so many directions and walking is the one place where I can give myself a shot of happiness. My day just seems to lighten the moment I put my shoes on and start moving. Ever since I've been walking I have found I am a better wife, mother and friend. I'm more patient, content and compassionate and ever since I've been walking my work stress has dramatically changed. Home, family, work, life, everything really just seems to be so much better when I walk."

—Jasmine, 35, Mother Of Two and Entrepreneur

Many of our Walking 4 Wellness clients have realized walking isn't just to get in physical shape—it's one of the greatest treatments for our emotional and mental well-being. We like to say, "motion affects emotion." Walking is one of the best ways to reduce your stress, anxiety and depression, helping you feel good, happy, content and joyful. Give yourself the shot and gift of happiness by taking a mental break daily. Your heart, mind and spirit will thank you!

When we have support, life is much more meaningful, richer, happier and altogether better. Fitness is no different.

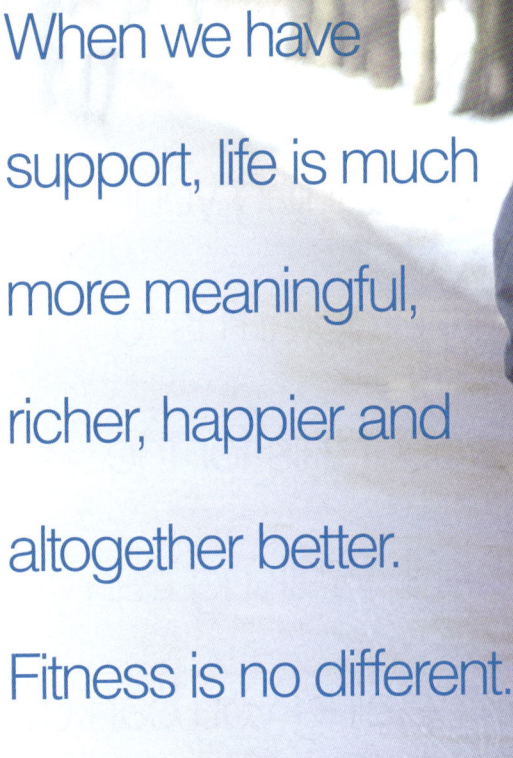

Walking 4 Living Well

One of the best perspectives to have when beginning your walking program is to think about this for the long haul. Walking can be something you can do for the rest of your life.

6 Get As Much Information As You Can!

"I read a book about the benefits of walking and I was sold! It not only made a huge impact on my health and fitness, but it also made me hungry to learn more. I read anything I can get my hands on about health, fitness and wellness. I subscribed to a few magazines that continue to motivate me to this day. Magazines like; *Walking, Shape* and *Prevention* are three of my favorites to inspire and motivate me to continue to walk and live well. The success stories help me to believe I can do it too!"

—Lani, 35, Hotel Administrator

Lani and many others have become life long students of health and wellness and are reaping the benefits of information, inspiration and motivation to keep on moving. In Chapter 7, you'll find a number of recommended resources to help you continue to learn more and encourage you to experience the power of walking.

7 Make Walking Fun

"I think the best tip I could share with someone who wants to start and maintain a consistent walking program is to make it fun! Like anything in life, I have found if you are having fun, you'll want to do it more. If it is a bore you'll find a way to quit. I have found being a kid again and finding the wonder in walking is one of the main reasons I do it. It makes me feel young again and I've been doing it for years now!"

—Jim, 65, Manufacturing Manager

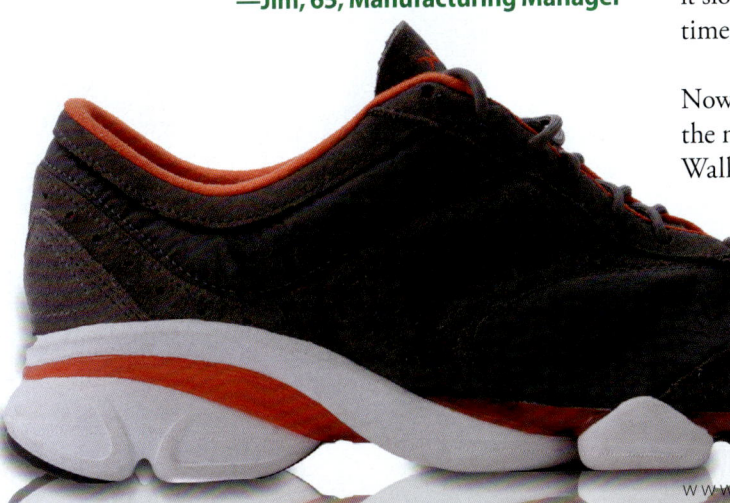

Making walking fun, or fitness for that matter, is one of the best ways to ensure your success. Go back to fifth grade and think of all the fun ways you found to entertain yourself when walking to school, to your friends' house or to a park and add them to your walking. How about trying to walk and…

- ✓ Sing
- ✓ Laugh
- ✓ Skip
- ✓ Imagine
- ✓ Jump
- ✓ Dream
- ✓ Make it an adventure (walk in different neighborhoods, terrain or trails)
- ✓ Be mindful of your surroundings (trees, birds, wildlife)

8 Be In It For Life

"The best advice I can give to someone who wants to start walking and keep walking is to remember it's not a race, but a lifelong journey of small steady steps to a healthier you. If you focus on one day at a time, then you'll find your weeks, months and years healthier and healthier!"

—Bob, 75, Retiree

One of the best perspectives to have when beginning your walking program is to think about this for the long haul. Walking can be something you can do for the rest of your life. So no need to rush or go crazy, you can take it slow and progress each and every week or month. In time, you'll be amazed at the life you have created.

Now that you've read some tried and true tips, let's go to the next chapter and put it all together and create your Walking 4 Wellness program!

To learn more about investing in a good pair of shoes, see page 29!

Chapter 7

Win 4 Today:
Putting It All Together

Designing Your
Walking 4 Wellness Plan

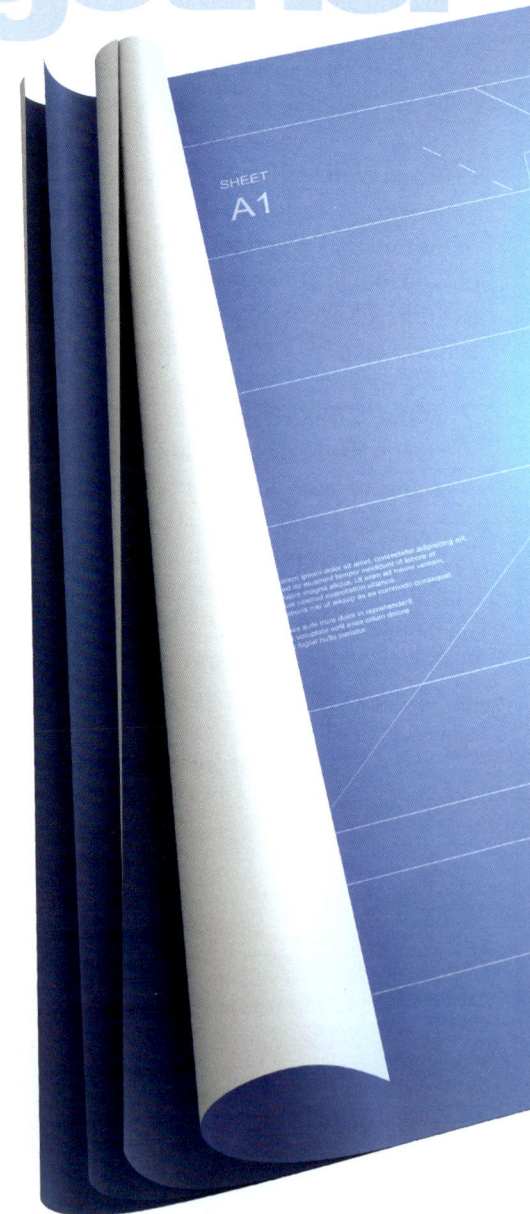

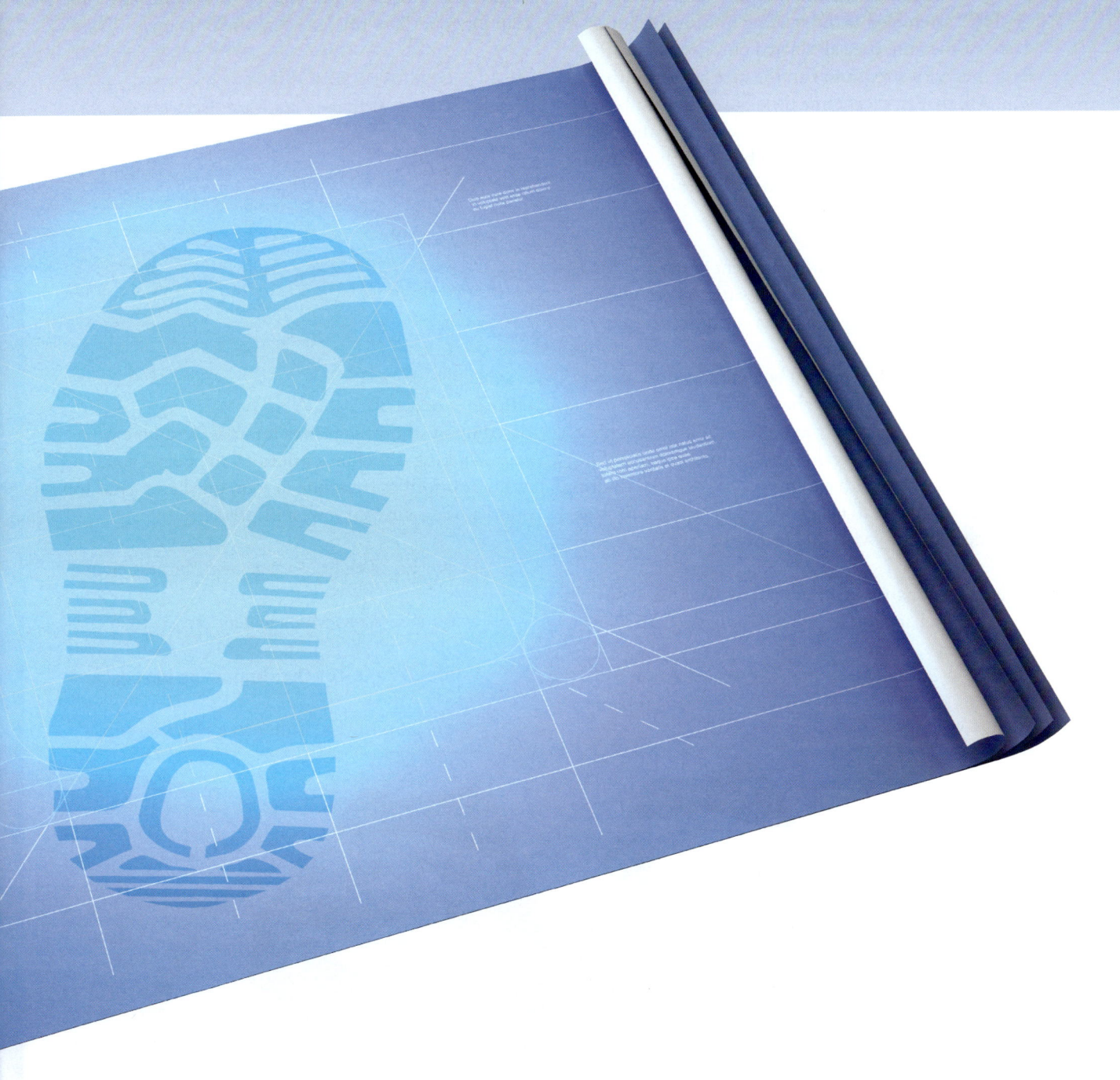

Win 4 Today:
Putting It All Together

A few years ago, at the Seattle Special Olympics, nine contestants, all physically or mentally disabled, assembled at the starting line for the 100-yard dash. At the gun, they all started out, not exactly in a dash, but with a relish to run the race to the finish and win. All, that is, except one little boy who stumbled on the asphalt, tumbled over a couple of times, and began to cry. The other eight heard the boy cry. They slowed down and looked back. Then they all turned around and went back.

One girl with Down's Syndrome bent down and kissed him and said: "This will make it better." Then all nine linked arms and walked together to the finish line.

You may have picked up this book to make changes in your own life. Or you may have been motivated to read this book to help a family member, friend or neighbor realize their personal health and wellness dreams. Or maybe you are a health and fitness professional desiring to make an impact to help your business, organization or company get moving and finish the race.

Whatever your goals are, you'll find a Walking 4 Wellness plan in this chapter to help you or others you know win.

It's time to put it all together. The worksheet on the following pages will help you craft a successful plan to Walk 4 Wellness.

Walking 4 Wellness Plan

Take a few minutes to put together a Walking 4 Wellness plan for you, those you love or your company.

Step 1—Determine Your **WHO:**

This Walking 4 Wellness Plan is for: (select one)

▶ Me

▶ My family

▶ My friends

▶ My company

▶ Other: _____

Step 2—Designate your **WHAT:**

Based upon who your plan is for, now designate what your Walking 4 Wellness priorities are. Select your wellness priorities from one to four, one being your top priority and four your lowest priority.

____ Body (Ex: Weight Management, Fitness etc.)

____ Mind (Ex: Stress Management etc.)

____ Career & Finances (Ex: Improving job goals)

____ Heart & Spirit (Ex: Enhancing Relationships)

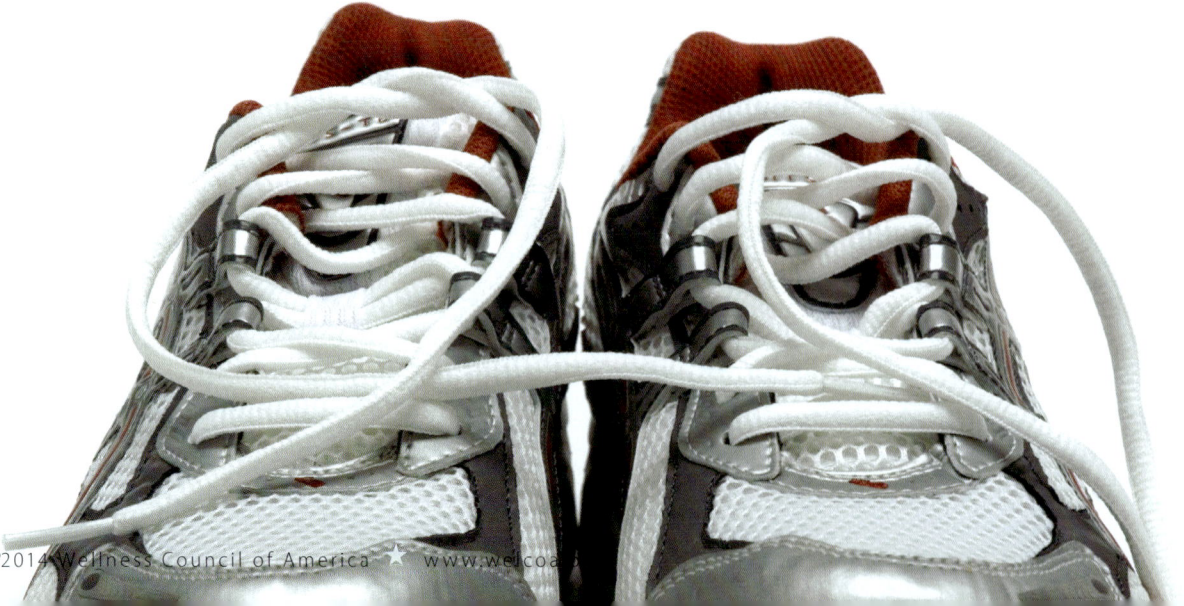

Step 3—Describe Your **WHERE:**

Where would you like to see changes? Describe in each Walking 4 Wellness "area" the changes you would like to see one year from now. For example, if you are personally interested in losing weight, you may want to write down, "One year from today I will lose _____ number of pounds." Or if you are designing your Walking 4 Wellness plan for your company, you may describe it like this, "We will enroll 30% of our company in a Walking 4 Wellness campaign and reduce 10% of our participants' body weight one year from the program start date." To help with this step, be as specific as you can:

Body:_____

_____

_____

Mind:_____

_____

_____

Career & Finances: _____

_____

_____

Heart & Spirit: _____

_____

_____

Win 4 Today: Putting It All Together

Step 4—Determine **WHEN** And **HOW LONG** Your Walking 4 Wellness Challenge Will Be:

Based upon who you are designing this plan for, your priorities and goals, determine your start date, and how many weeks you would like your Walking 4 Wellness Challenge to be:

▶ Start Date: _____

  – 4 Weeks

  – 8 Weeks

  – 12 Weeks

  – 16 Weeks

▶ End Date: _____

For example, if you'd like to lose weight and improve your spiritual health you can create an eight-week challenge,

>   4 Weeks of Body Walking
>
> +   4 Weeks of Heart/Spirit Walking
> _____
> =   8 Week Waking 4 Wellness Challenge

Or, for those of you in charge of designing your health and wellness services or offering health and fitness programs for your employees you may want to design a 12-week challenge to help employees improve their Body, Mind and Financial health. You can provide monthly lunch and learn sessions on each aspect of Walking 4 Wellness and create a 12-week challenge. Your 12-week Walking 4 Wellness Challenge may look something like this:

Date	Walking 4 Wellness Focus	Education	Support
January	4 Weeks Body	Lunch & Learn	Walking Groups
February	4 Weeks Mind	Lunch & Learn	Walking Groups
March	4 Weeks Career/Finances	Lunch & Learn	Walking Groups
	= 12 Week Challenge		

The possibilities are endless. You can create a year-long Walking 4 Wellness campaign, focusing on one of the wellness areas presented in this book as your quarterly theme and offer walking groups and incentives prizes for each wellness area completed:

Date	Walking 4 Wellness Focus	Support	Incentives
January	12 Weeks Body	Walking Groups	Resistance bands
April	12 Weeks Mind	Walking Groups	MP3
July	12 Weeks Career/Finances	Walking Groups	Voom
October	12 Weeks Heart/Spirit	Walking Groups	CDs
	= 1 Year Campaign		

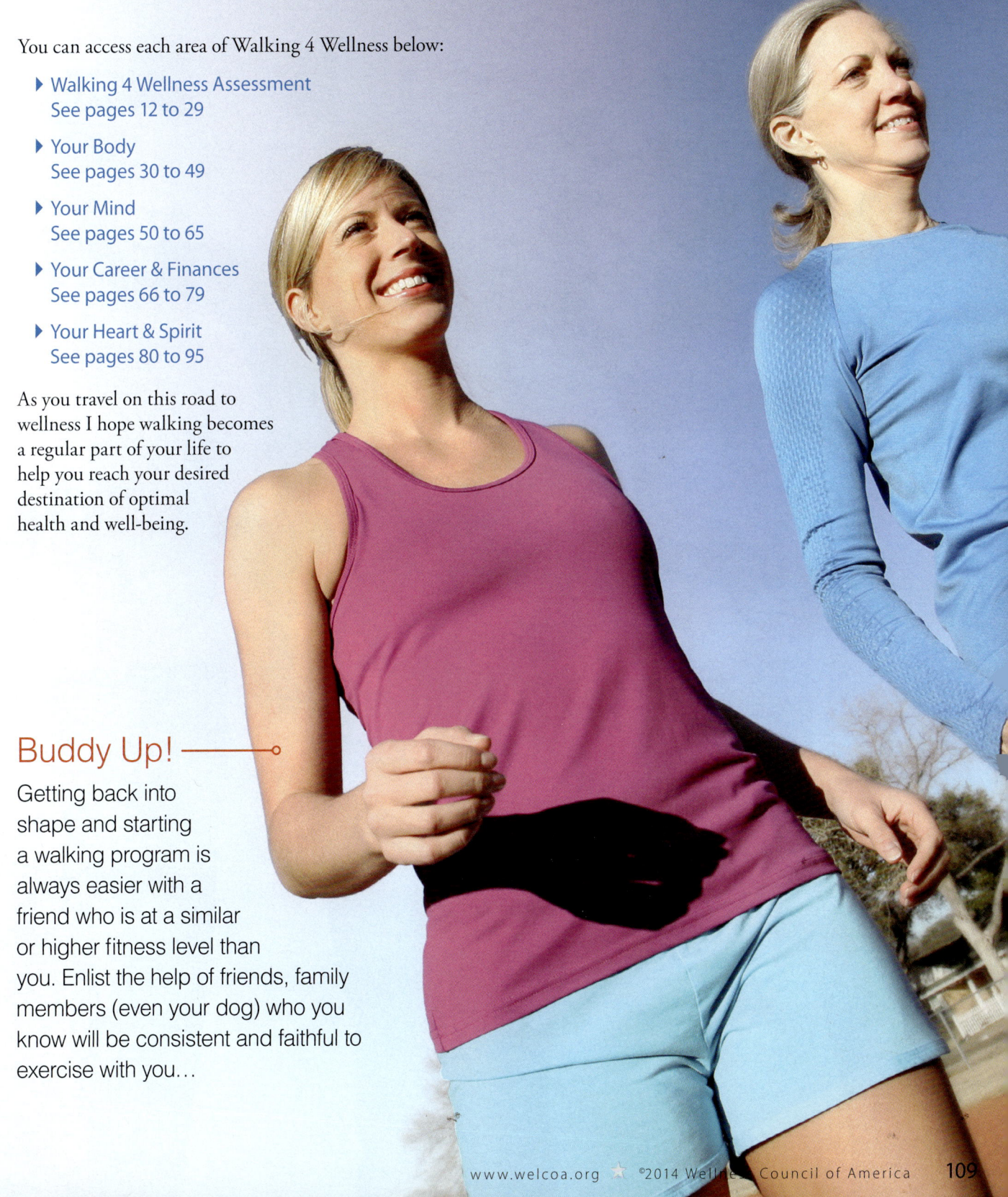

You can access each area of Walking 4 Wellness below:

▶ **Walking 4 Wellness Assessment**
See pages 12 to 29

▶ **Your Body**
See pages 30 to 49

▶ **Your Mind**
See pages 50 to 65

▶ **Your Career & Finances**
See pages 66 to 79

▶ **Your Heart & Spirit**
See pages 80 to 95

As you travel on this road to wellness I hope walking becomes a regular part of your life to help you reach your desired destination of optimal health and well-being.

Buddy Up!

Getting back into shape and starting a walking program is always easier with a friend who is at a similar or higher fitness level than you. Enlist the help of friends, family members (even your dog) who you know will be consistent and faithful to exercise with you…

In Summary:
Walking 4 Wellness

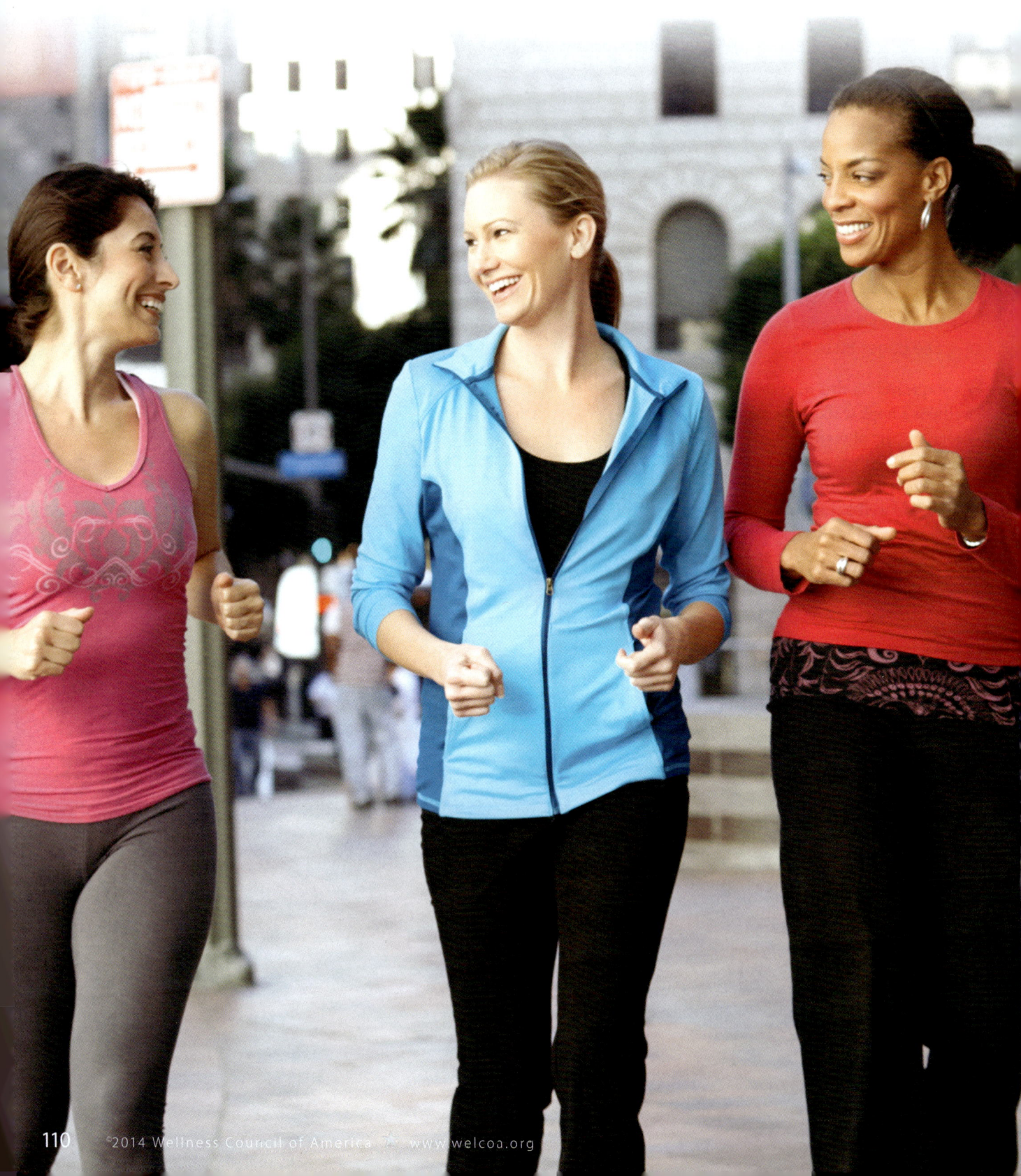

As you travel on this road to wellness I hope walking becomes a regular part of your life to help you reach your desired dreams and destination of optimal health and well-being.

Just remember along your journey to:

Remind Yourself To Win Today! Forget about yesterday and try not to think about tomorrow. Focus your attention on what you can do today. Ask yourself, "How can I win today?" No matter what your previous experiences or attempts to change your fitness habits in the past have been, remind yourself today is a new day. Begin by taking one step and one day at a time!

Plan Your Walking! Good walking and exercise habits happen because we make them happen. Schedule "non-negotiable" appointments to take a walk—even if it is just five or 10 minutes. Soon enough, your regular walks will be something you cherish, protect and look forward to!

Stop And Smell The Roses! Be sure to stop and congratulate yourself as you accomplish even the smallest of goals. Soon you'll realize your dreams, making Walking 4 Wellness not just what you do—but who you are.

Share Your Story With Us And With Others! One of the best ways to make Walking 4 Wellness a regular part of your life is to share your story with others. Make it a point to share with those you love, those in your company or community how to Walk 4 Wellness. By sharing your story you'll not only support your efforts, you'll inspire those around you.

Win Today
I'd love to hear how you are Walking 4 Wellness. Go to my website, **wintodaywellness.com** and tell us what has worked for you and how you "won today."

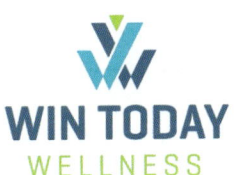

My website is filled with inspiring stories of individuals who are striving to win each and every day. Come join us and receive ongoing encouragement, inspiration and support to help you make Walking 4 Wellness a reality for you. Here you'll find:

▸ Proven fitness tips to help you get fit and stay fit

▸ Inspiring Win Today interviews

▸ Videos

▸ Webinars

▸ Body, mind, heart and spirit resources

▸ FAQ's and more…

You can also get daily coaching and tips by joining me on Twitter at **@coachseanfoy**

We'd love to hear from you! Here's wishing you, your family and your company the greatest of success today and always as you Walk 4 Wellness!

Win today! All the best!

Sean Foy, MA

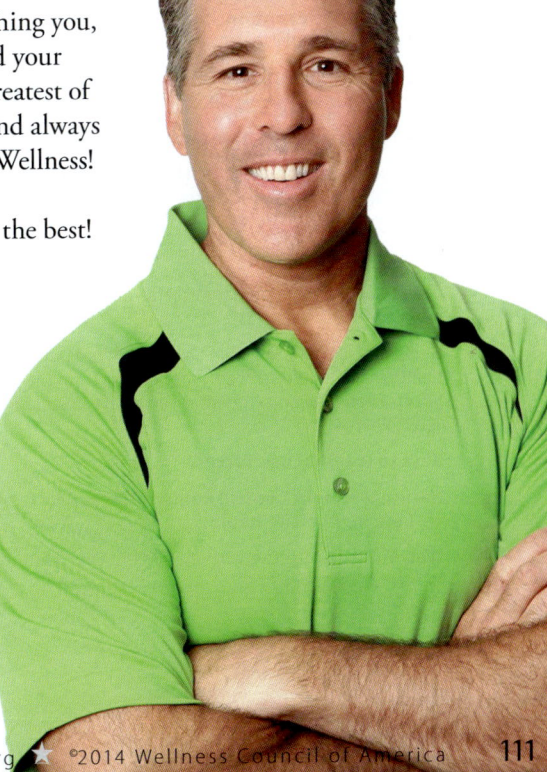

References/Resources

Introduction

Snow White and the Seven Dwarfs. Treasure Box of Children's Stories. Platt & Munk Co., 1922.

Walt Disney's Snow White and the Seven Dwarfs. Story adapted by Jane Werner. Illus. by the Walt Disney Studio adapted by Campbell Grant. Racine, WI: Golden Press, 1952.

Well Being-The Five Essential Elements. Rath, Tom, Harter, Jim. (2010). Gallup Press: New York, NY.

Chapter 1: Four Simple Steps To Walk This Way

80-year-old Japanese man becomes oldest to climb Mount Everest. (See: http://www.cnn.com/2013/05/23/world/asia/nepal-everest-record)

Walking 4 Wellness Assessment:

Well Being-The Five Essential Elements. Rath, Tom, Harter, Jim. (2010). Gallup Press: New York, NY.

See: **http://wellness.ucr.edu/seven_dimensions.html** and also **http://definitionofwellness.com/index.html**

Walk of Weight, Stanten, Michele (2010). Prevention; Rodale Inc. New York, NY

Fitness Walking for Dummies, Neporent, Liz (2000), IDG Books Worldwide, California

Duke University: http://www.dukehealth.org/health_library/health_articles/finding_the_right_running_shoe

Chapter 2: Walking 4 Your Body

The Benefits of Physical Activity and Exercise; Centers for Disease Control and Prevention; (See http://www.cdc.gov/physicalactivity/everyone/health/)

U.S. Dept. of Health and Human Services. 2008 Physical Activity Guidelines for Americans, 2008

The American Heart Association:

http://www.heart.org/HEARTORG/GettingHealthy/PhysicalActivity/StartWalking/Physical-activity-improves-quality-of-life_UCM_307977_Article.jsp

Harvard University:

(See: http://www.hsph.harvard.edu/nutritionsource/staying-active-full-story/)

Nelson ME, Rejeski WJ, Blair SN, et al. Physical activity and public health in older adults: recommendation from the American College of Sports Medicine and the American Heart Association. Circulation. 2007; 116:1094-105.

Keys to Weight Loss Success:

National Weight Control Registry Research (See: http://www.nwcr.ws/Research/default.htm)

Web MD (See http://www.webmd.com/diet/features/4-keys-weight-loss-success?page=3)

Klem ML, Wing RR, McGuire MT, Seagle HM & Hill JO (1997). A descriptive study of individuals successful at long-term maintenance of substantial weight loss. American Journal of Clinical Nutrition, 66, 239-246.

Wyatt HR, Grunwald OK, Mosca CL, Klem ML, Wing RR, Hill JO. (2002). Long-term weight loss and breakfast in subjects in the National Weight Control Registry. Obesity Research, 10, 78-82.

Wing RR & Hill JO. (2001). Successful weight loss maintenance. Annual Review of Nutrition, 21, 323-341.

Thomas JG, Wing RR. (2009). Maintenance of long-term weight loss. Medicine & Health Rhode Island 92, 2, 56-57

V.A. Victoria A. Catenacci1, et al., "Physical Activity patterns in the National Weight Control Registry," Obesity 16 (2008); 153-61

The Complete Guide to Walking, New and Revised: For Health, Weight Loss and Fitness (Connecticut; The Lyons Press, 2008)

Walk of Weight, Stanten, Michele (2010). Prevention; Rodale Inc. New York, NY

Chapter 3: Walking 4 Your Mind

Weir, K. (2011). "The Exercise Effect." Monitor on Psychology, American Psychological Association, 42(11), p. 48.

Peluso MA, Andrade LH. Physical activity and mental health: the association between exercise and mood. Clinics. 2005;60:61–70.

Callaghan P. Exercise: a neglected intervention in mental health care? J Psychiatr Ment Health Nurs. 2004;11:476–483.

Mayo Clinic: (See: http://www.mayoclinic.com/health/depression-and-exercise/MH00043)

The Psychology of Exercise: (See: http://www.ideafit.com/fitness-library/psychology-exercise-1)

Sichel, D. & Driscoll, J. (1999). Women's Moods: What Every Woman Must Know About Hormones, The Brain, and Emotional Health, pp. 113-114.

Cohen, S. and Williamson, G. Perceived Stress in a Probability Sample of the United States. Spacapan, S. and Oskamp, S. (Eds.) The Social Psychology of Health. Newbury Park, CA: Sage, 1988.

Cohen, S., Kamarck, T., & Mermelstein, R. (1983). A global measure of perceived stress. Journal of Health and Social Behavior, 24, 385-396.

Mellin, Laurel. (2010)"Wired for Joy!: A Revolutionary Method for Creating Happiness from Within." Hay House, Inc.

Dr. Marc Siegel, (See: www.washingtonpost.com/wp-dyn/content/article/2007/01/05/AR2007010501398.html)

Berk L, Tan S, Fry W, Napier B, Lee J, Hubbard R, et al. Neuroendocrine and stress hormone changes during mirthful laughter. The American Journal of the Medical Sciences 1989;298:391–6

Cousins, Norman, Anatomy of an illness as Perceived by the Patient, New York: Norton, 1979.

Laugh Scientist: (See: http://mentalfloss.com/article/30329/lab-worlds-leading-laugh-scientist)

Dr. Madan Kataria and Laughter Yoga (See: http://www.wikihow.com/Do-Laughter-Yoga and http://laughteryoga.org/english/laughteryoga)

Dogs increase walking (See: http://www.ava.com.au/mediarelease/pets-provide-powerful-benefits-people

Chapter 4: Walking For Your Career & Finances

7 Benefits of Exercise, Mayo Clinic (See http://www.mayoclinic.com/health/exercise/HQ01676)

The benefits of physical activity. Centers for Disease Control and Prevention. http://www.cdc.gov/physicalactivity/everyone/health/index.html. Accessed July 5, 2011.

Economic Benefits of Regular Exercise (See: www.healthclubs.com and http://www.resultsthegym.com/Uploads/file/EconomicsOfRegularExercise.pdf)

U.S. Dept. of Health and Human Services. 2008 Physical Activity Guidelines for Americans. 2008.

Dr. Ronald Davis on Exercise: Exercise is Medicine. A Newsletter Promoting the Benefits of Physical Activity. Volume 1, Spring 2008.

Jacobson, B. and S. Aldana. Relationship Between Frequency of Aerobic Activity and Illness-Related Absenteeismin a Large Employee Sample. Journal of Occupational and Environmental Medicine. December 2001; 43(12); 1019-1025.

Burton,W. et al. The Association of Health Riskswith On-the-Job Productivity. Journal of Occupational and Environmental Medicine. August 2005. 47(8):769-777.

Fitness That Works, Foy, Sean (2011) WELCOA Publishing, Omaha NE.

Chapter 5: Walking For Your Heart & Spirit

Ornish D. Love & Survival: The Scientific Basis for the Healing Power of Intimacy. New York: HarperCollins, 1998

Mendes de Leon CF. Why do friendships matter for survival? Journal of Epidemiology and Community Health. 2005;59:537.

Mellor D. Need for belonging, relationship satisfaction, loneliness, and life satisfaction. Personality and Individual Differences. 2008;45:213.

Peter C. Hill and Eric M. Butter (1995) "The Role of Religion in Promoting Physical Health." Journal of Psychology and Christianity 14 (2): 141-155)

Rosemarie Kobau1, Joseph Sniezek, et al., "Well-Being Assessment: An Evaluation of Well-Being Scales for Public Health and Population Estimates of Well-Being among US Adults," *Applied Psychology: Health and Well-Being*, Nov. 2010, 272-297

Matthews DA, Koenig HG, Thoresen C, Friedman R. Physical health. In Larson DB, Swyers JP, McCullough ME, eds. Scientific Research on Spirituality and Health. Rockville, MD: National Institute for Healthcare Research; 1998.

Jean Pollack, "What Is My Life's Purpose?" Psychology Today, Sept. 14, 2011,

(See: http://www.psychologytoday.com/blog/creativity-way-life/201109/what-is-my-lifes-purpose)

Self Hugging (See: www.psychologytoday.com/blog/the-science-willpower/201105/hugging-yourself-reduces-physical-pain)

Gallace A, Torta DM, Moseley GL, & Iannetti GD (2011) The analgesic effect of crossing the arms. Pain 152(6):1418-23.

Eight Hugs a day keeps the doctor away: (See: (http://positivepsychologynews.com/news/emiliya-zhivotovskaya/2012032321636)

Loved and cared for (See: http://www.psychologytoday.com/blog/stronger-the-broken-places/201201/the-real-key-good-health)

Social Networks and Health. *MIT researcher finds that social networks influence health behaviors.* (See: www. web.mit.edu)

The 10-Minute Total Body Breakthrough, Foy, Sean (2009) Workman Publishing, New York, NY

Chapter 6: Walking 4 Living Well

Dallas Bed rest story

McGuire DK, Levine BD, Williamson JW, et al. A 30-Year Follow-Up of the Dallas Bed Rest and Training Study. Circulation. 2001;104:1350.

Chapter 7: Win 4 Today

Throughout this book, I recommend various products and tools to help you Walk 4 Wellness. Many of the products and tools are available at **www.wintodaywellness.com** and also at local sporting good stores or online. Feel free to shop around to find the best price and product to meet your needs.

Walking 4 Wellness Web Links:

Adidas (www.adidas.com)

Aerobics and Fitness Association of America (www.afaa.com)

American Academy of Orthopedic Surgeons (wwaaos.org)

American Council on Exercise (www.acefitness.org)

American Podiatric Medical Association (www.apma.org)

American Alliance for Health, Physical Education, Recreation and Dance (www.aahperd.org)

American College of Sports Medicine (www.acsm.org)

American Journal of Health Promotion (www.ajhp.com)

Asics (www.asicsamerica.com)

Idea Health and Fitness Association (www.ideafit.com)

International Health, Racquet & Sports club Association (IHRSA) consumer web site: (www.healthclubs.com)

Landice Treadmills (www.landice.com)

Let's Move: (www.letsmove.gov)

National Strength & Conditioning Association: (www.nsca-lift.org)

National Institute of Health (www.nih.gov)

New Balance Athletic Shoe (www.newbalance.com)

Nike (www.nike.com)

Office of the Surgeon General (www.surgeongeneral.gov)

Polar Heart Rate Monitor (www.polar.com)

Physical Activity Guidelines (www.cdc.gov/physicalactivity)

Presidents Council On Physical Fitness & Sports (www.fitness.gov)

Reebok (www.reebok.com)

Saucony (www.saucony.com)

Special Olympics International: (www.specialolympics.org)

Wellness Council of America (www.welcoa.org)

YMCA and YWCA: (www.ymca.net and www.ywca.org)

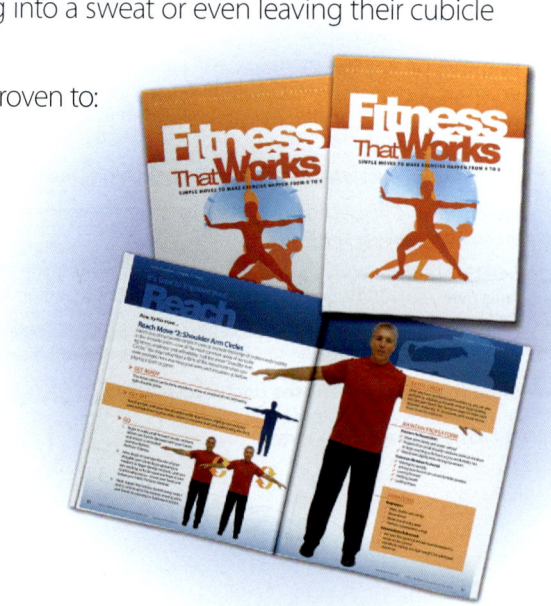

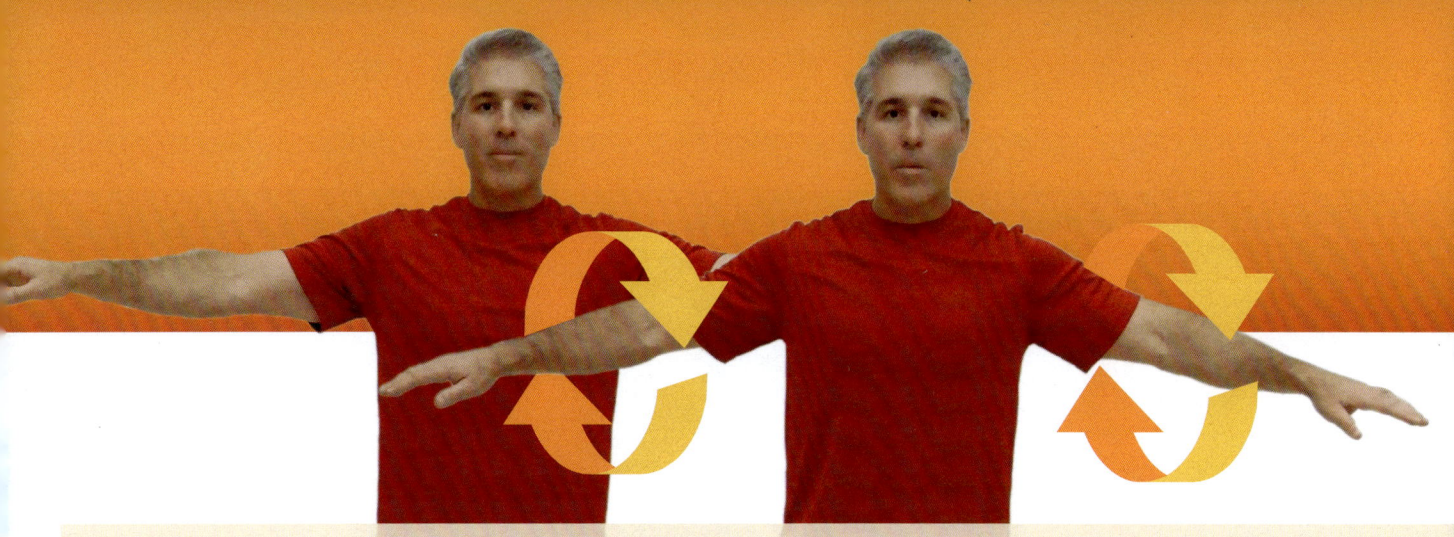

"By leveraging simple moves that have HUGE payoff, Sean Foy's *Fitness That Works* will impact you and your organization in important ways. Not only will you become healthier, you'll also become happier, more productive and more engaged."

David Hunnicutt, PhD
President, WELCOA

Fitness That Works…
The perfect incentive for your employees!

> ➤ Health Fairs

> ➤ HRA Incentives

> ➤ New Employee Orientation

> ➤ Lunch n' Learns

> ➤ Behavior Change Campaigns

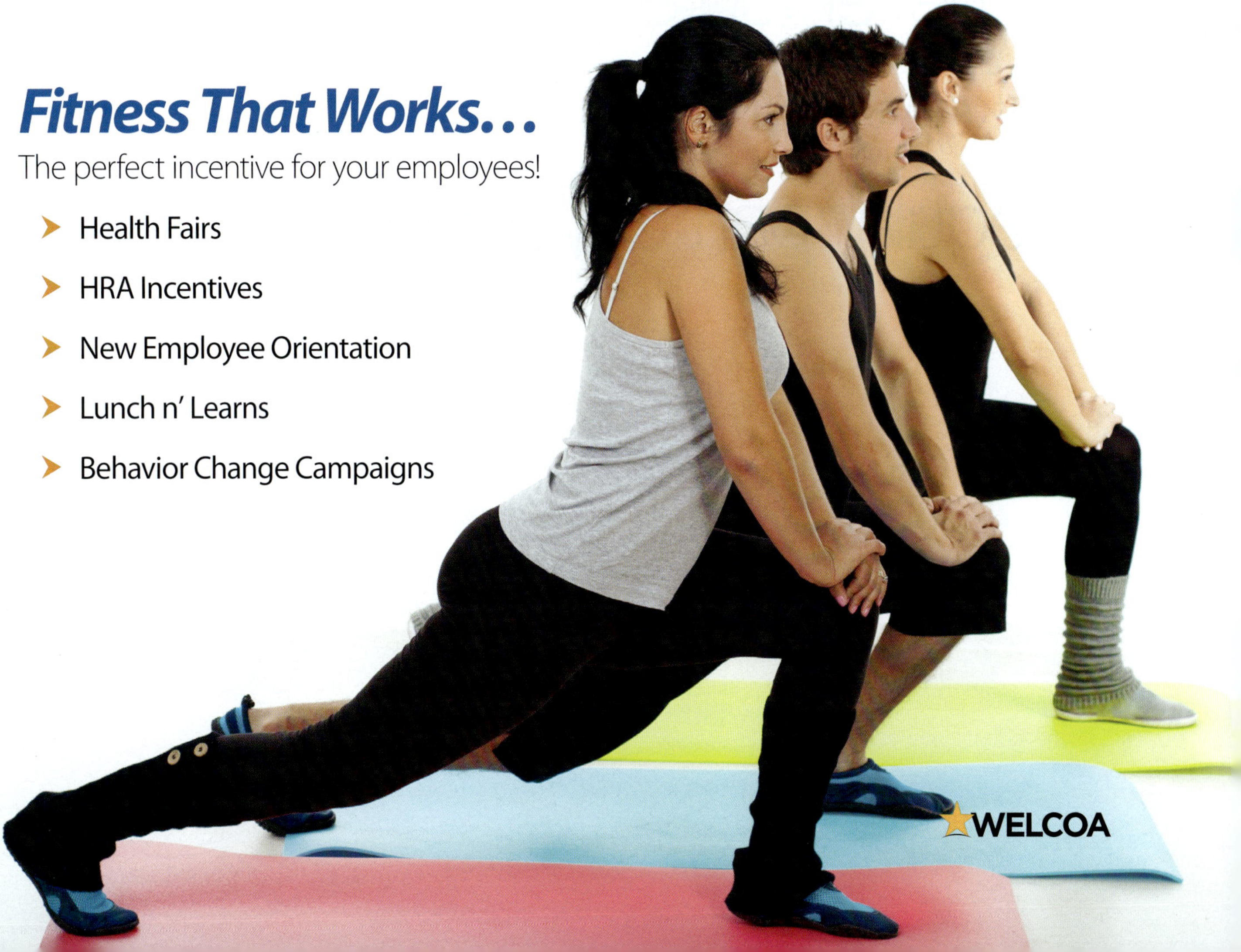

★WELCOA

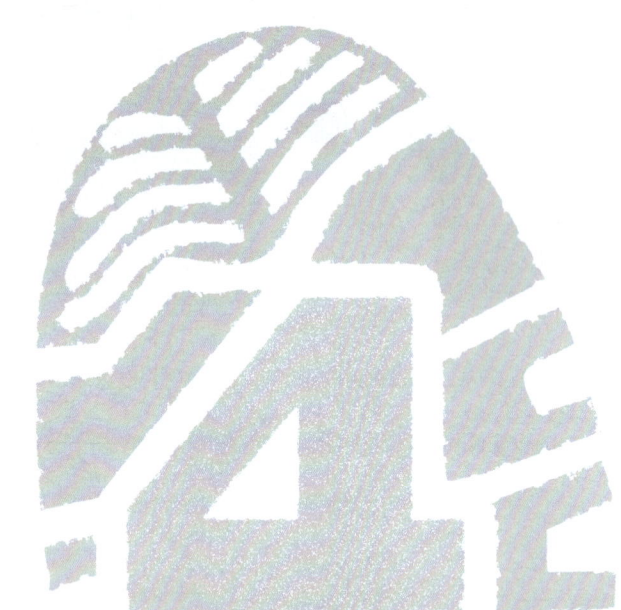

It is never too early or too late to make walking and physical activity a regular part of your life!